I0473305

Get ahead!
Medicine
300 SBAs for Finals

Get ahead! Medicine: 300 SBAs for Finals, fully revised and updated in this second edition, provides invaluable revision for all medical students preparing for finals exams through plentiful practice questions, similar to those you can expect in the real exam. It features:

- 300 SBA questions written in a similar style to the Medical Schools Council Assessment Alliance (MSC-AA) bank
- Examples of harder stems for students aiming for honours
- Eponymous details and derivatives for added interest
- Full explanatory answers including succinct subject summaries

Covering the entire syllabus in a clear and comprehensive style, this book provides reliable and effective revision practice to help you pass your final medical exams.

AUTHORS

Hiruni Jayasena is a Senior Lecturer in Clinical Medicine at General Sir John Kotelawala Defence University (KDU) and an Honorary Consultant Gastroenterologist and Hepatologist at the University Hospital KDU, Boralesgamuwa, Sri Lanka.

Benjamin R.T. Wood is a Registrar in Plastic Surgery and a Member of the Faculty of Surgical Trainers of the Royal College of Surgeons of Edinburgh, UK.

Marilena Giannoudi is an Academic Clinical Lecturer in Cardiology at the University of Leeds and a Registrar in Cardiology and General Internal Medicine at Leeds Teaching Hospitals, UK.

SERIES EDITOR

Saran Shantikumar is a Consultant and Associate Clinical Professor in Public Health at the University of Warwick, UK.

Get ahead!

Series Editor: Saran Shantikumar

Get ahead!

Medicine
300 SBAs for Finals

Second edition

Hiruni Jayasena
Benjamin R.T. Wood
Marilena Giannoudi

Series Editor
Saran Shantikumar

CRC Press
Taylor & Francis Group
Boca Raton London New York

CRC Press is an imprint of the
Taylor & Francis Group, an **informa** business

Second edition published 2026
by CRC Press
2385 NW Executive Center Drive, Suite 320, Boca Raton FL 33431

and by CRC Press
4 Park Square, Milton Park, Abingdon, Oxon, OX14 4RN

CRC Press is an imprint of Taylor & Francis Group, LLC

© 2026 Hiruni Jayasena, Benjamin R.T. Wood, and Marilena Giannoudi

This book contains information obtained from authentic and highly regarded sources. While all reasonable efforts have been made to publish reliable data and information, neither the author[s] nor the publisher can accept any legal responsibility or liability for any errors or omissions that may be made. The publishers wish to make clear that any views or opinions expressed in this book by individual editors, authors or contributors are personal to them and do not necessarily reflect the views/opinions of the publishers. The information or guidance contained in this book is intended for use by medical, scientific or health-care professionals and is provided strictly as a supplement to the medical or other professional's own judgement, their knowledge of the patient's medical history, relevant manufacturer's instructions and the appropriate best practice guidelines. Because of the rapid advances in medical science, any information or advice on dosages, procedures or diagnoses should be independently verified. The reader is strongly urged to consult the relevant national drug formulary and the drug companies' and device or material manufacturers' printed instructions, and their websites, before administering or utilizing any of the drugs, devices or materials mentioned in this book. This book does not indicate whether a particular treatment is appropriate or suitable for a particular individual. Ultimately it is the sole responsibility of the medical professional to make his or her own professional judgements, so as to advise and treat patients appropriately. The authors and publishers have also attempted to trace the copyright holders of all material reproduced in this publication and apologize to copyright holders if permission to publish in this form has not been obtained. If any copyright material has not been acknowledged please write and let us know so we may rectify in any future reprint.

Except as permitted under U.S. Copyright Law, no part of this book may be reprinted, reproduced, transmitted, or utilized in any form by any electronic, mechanical, or other means, now known or hereafter invented, including photocopying, microfilming, and recording, or in any information storage or retrieval system, without written permission from the publishers.

For permission to photocopy or use material electronically from this work, access www.copyright.com or contact the Copyright Clearance Center, Inc. (CCC), 222 Rosewood Drive, Danvers, MA 01923, 978-750-8400. For works that are not available on CCC please contact mpkbookspermissions@tandf.co.uk

Trademark notice: Product or corporate names may be trademarks or registered trademarks and are used only for identification and explanation without intent to infringe.

ISBN: 978-1-041-09049-6 (hbk)
ISBN: 978-1-041-09047-2 (pbk)
ISBN: 978-1-003-64822-2 (ebk)

DOI: 10.1201/9781003648222

Typeset in Minion Pro
by Apex CoVantage, LLC

Contents

Acknowledgements

The authors of this second edition and the series editor wish to acknowledge and thank the authors of the first edition, Benjamin McNeillis, Rhian James, Ai Ling Koh and Tim Sparkes, upon whose work this second edition draws.

Practice paper 1: Questions

1. Acute coronary syndrome

In the treatment of acute coronary syndrome (ACS), which of the following statements is FALSE?

A Heparin should be given alongside anti-platelet therapy in the acute setting

B Give 75 mg aspirin stat

C Clopidogrel 300 mg stat is given as the second anti-platelet agent

D Hypotension, asthma and bradycardia are the main contraindicators to beta blockade

E Patients will likely continue taking a statin, beta-blocker and angiotensin-converting enzyme (ACE) inhibitor on discharge home

2. Obstructive renal impairment

Which of the following is NOT a potential cause of obstructive renal impairment?

A Benign prostatic hypertrophy

B Recurrent kidney stones

C Retroperitoneal fibrosis

D Schistosomiasis

E Systemic sclerosis

3. Management of skin lesions

A 60-year-old man who works for an oil company presents with a growing lesion on the temple. It bled once when he knocked it. On examination, the lesion is 8 mm in diameter and is a flat, mildly erythematous patch with a few scales and a larger keratotic horn in the centre. There are no other lesions on inspection of his skin and no personal or family history of skin cancer.

Which of the following is the most appropriate management plan?

A Cryotherapy

B Curettage

C Excisional biopsy

D Topical 5-fluorouracil

E Radiotherapy

DOI: 10.1201/9781003648222-1

4. Chest X-ray

A 68-year-old man who is recently diagnosed with lung cancer is admitted to the emergency department with acute shortness of breath. A chest X-ray shows a right upper zone (RUZ) collapse.

What do you expect to find on examination?

	Trachea	Percussion	Auscultation
A	Deviated to right	Dull RUZ	Reduced breath sounds
B	Deviated to right	Dull RUZ	Wheeze
C	Deviated to right	Resonant RUZ	Reduced breath sounds
D	Deviated to left	Dull RUZ	Reduced breath sounds
E	Deviated to left	Resonant RUZ	Wheeze

5. Headaches

A 68-year-old woman presents to her GP with headaches and visual disturbance. She has also noticed that she gets an itchy rash when she gets out of a hot bath. On examination she has a ruddy complexion and a palpable spleen. Her only previous medical history is gout. Initial blood tests reveal a raised packed red cell volume with a raised red cell mass, along with a raised white cell count and thrombocytosis.

What is the most likely diagnosis?

A Chronic myeloid leukaemia
B Lymphoma
C Migraine with aura
D Polycythaemia rubra vera
E Soap allergy

6. Chronic obstructive pulmonary disease

A 45-year-old man who is a heavy smoker has chronic obstructive pulmonary disease (COPD). He has no other past medical history, including no asthmatic features to his disease. He has seen the GP today, as he feels his breathing has been getting progressively worse over the last few weeks, and he is wheezy and is coughing more frequently. He currently takes PRN salbutamol but reports using it more frequently over the last few weeks. His FEV_1 on this occasion is 35%. He is talking in full sentences, and observations are stable with no sign of infection.

Which of the following is the next step in management?

A Add in PRN ipratropium
B Add in inhaled corticosteroids
C Add in a long-acting beta-agonist (salmeterol) with a long-acting muscarinic antagonist (tiotropium)
D Switch salbutamol for ipratropium PRN
E Admit to hospital for acute COPD exacerbation management

7. Management of asthma

A 35-year-old woman is admitted to hospital with quick-onset shortness of breath. She has a past medical history of asthma. Her observations include a pulse rate 120 bpm, blood pressure 100/72 mmHg, respiratory rate 30/min and SaO_2 88% on room air. On examination, she appears to be drowsy and exhausted. Her chest is quiet on auscultation. Arterial blood gases show pH 7.35, PaO_2 5.2 kPa, $PaCO_2$ 4.9 kPa and bicarbonate 24 mmol/L.

Which of the following would NOT be appropriate in the management of this case?

A High-flow oxygen
B High-dose nebulised beta-2 agonists
C Intravenous magnesium sulphate
D Leukotriene receptor antagonists
E Steroids

8. Collapse

A 19-year-old man has collapsed on the pitch whilst playing Sunday league football. He reports being normally fit and well, although he had a late night before the game attending a friend's birthday party, consuming large amounts of alcohol and not sleeping well. On examination his airway is clear, but he does seem a little agitated, and observations demonstrate a slight tachycardia of 105 bpm. He has never experienced anything like this before. There is no family history of similar events.

Which of the following is the most likely diagnosis?

A Carotid stenosis
B Hypertrophic obstructive cardiomyopathy (HOCM)
C Epileptic seizure
D Vasovagal
E Hypoglycaemia

9. Eczema versus psoriasis

A 31-year-old woman presents to your clinic with a year-long history of itchy, red, scaly lesions.

Which of the following would make you more likely to diagnose eczema rather than psoriasis?

A Associated nail changes
B History of distal interphalangeal joint pain and swelling
C Localised to flexures rather than extensors
D Well-demarcated lesions
E Occurring at the site of previous trauma

10. Diagnosis of multiple sclerosis

Which of the following best describes the MRI findings in multiple sclerosis?

A Cortical grey matter inflammatory lesions
B Longitudinally extensive transverse myelitis (more than three spinal segments)
C Periventricular white matter lesions matching the clinical picture
D Periventricular white matter lesions not necessarily matching the clinical picture
E White matter lesions exclusively in the cerebellum and brainstem

11. The multidisciplinary team

A 67-year-old man is discharged from hospital following an incision and drainage of a large abdominal wall abscess. He needs someone to help change his wound packing regularly; however, he is immobile and lives alone.

Which member of the multidisciplinary team would be most appropriate to help?

A District nurse   D Orthotist
B Health visitor   E Social worker
C Occupational therapist

12. Diagnosis of chest pain

A 27-year-old gentleman is seen in the accident and emergency department. He is 2 days post-open reduction and internal fixation of a left mid-shaft clavicle fracture he obtained following a fall. He is normally fit and well and reports he felt well in the immediate post-operative period; however, he felt pain in the left chest when sleeping last night. The pain is exacerbated by inspiration. Which investigation is the most appropriate primary investigation and likely to provide the diagnosis?

A ECG   D Full set of bloods including CRP
B CXR   E Intraoperative X-ray images
C Trauma CT

13. Risk factors for ischaemic heart disease

Which of the following reduces the risk of coronary artery disease?

A Smoking history of five cigarettes per day
B High low-density lipoprotein (LDL) cholesterol levels
C Hypertension
D Obesity
E Consuming 12 units of alcohol a week

14. Diagnosis of cough

A 29-year-old man presents to the emergency department with a 1-week history of non-productive cough, muscle aches, fever, vomiting and diarrhoea. His observations include temperature 38.4°C, pulse rate 105 bpm, blood pressure 110/76 mmHg and respiratory rate 22/min. On examination, his chest is clear to both auscultation and percussion. A chest X-ray shows bilateral lung basal infiltrates. The blood results show Na^+ 128 mmol/L, K^+ 4.0 mmol/L, urea 5.9 mmol/L, creatinine 130 μmol/L, albumin 26 g/L, ALT 106 IU/L and ALP 230 IU/L.

What is the most likely causative organism?

A *Chlamydia pneumoniae*
B *Mycoplasma pneumoniae*
C *Legionella pneumophila*
D *Staphylococcus aureus*
E *Streptococcus pneumoniae*

15. Diagnosis of vertigo

A 60-year-old man presents with a history of recurrent dizzy spells for the past 4 months, which occur daily. The dizzy spells last a few minutes and seem to occur if he moves his head, as a result of which he keeps his head as still as possible. The attacks are not associated with any deafness or tinnitus, and a neurological examination is entirely normal. You favour a diagnosis of benign paroxysmal positional vertigo.

Which of the following descriptions of findings on Hallpike's manoeuvre would confirm this diagnosis?

A Delayed onset (a few seconds) torsional nystagmus on descent facing both sides
B Delayed onset (a few seconds) torsional nystagmus on descent facing one side only
C Immediate torsional nystagmus on descent facing both sides
D Immediate torsional nystagmus on descent facing one side only
E No nystagmus on descent facing either side

16. Epistaxis

A 43-year-old man presents to his GP with a 3-month history of recurrent nosebleeds, mucosal bleeding, haemoptysis and recurrent sinusitis. Besides that, he also noticed that he has increasingly become short of breath. On examination, he had a nasal deformity, and chest auscultation revealed crackles in the left lower zone. A urine dipstick test showed microscopic haematuria.

Which of the following is the most likely diagnosis?

A Chronic myeloid leukaemia
B Chronic lymphocytic leukaemia
C Churg–Strauss syndrome (also known as eosinophilic granulomatosis with polyangiitis [EGPA])
D Goodpasture syndrome
E Granulomatosis with polyangiitis (GPA)

17. Diarrhoea

Following a protracted stay in hospital for the treatment of a severe chest infection, an 83-year-old man develops bloody diarrhoea.

What is the most likely cause?

A Adenocarcinoma of the bowel
B *Clostridium difficile* infection
C Norovirus infection
D *Salmonella* infection
E *Shigella* infection

18. Diagnosis of malaria

A 21-year-old student on an internship with the *Guardian* travel section has recently returned from a backpacking holiday in West Africa. For the last few days he has been having headaches, flu-like symptoms and muscle aches, and now he has started rigoring.

Which investigation should be performed to rule out malaria?

A Blood cultures
B *Falciparum* antigen dipstick test
C Liver biopsy
D One blood film
E Three thick and thin blood films on consecutive days

19. Electrocardiogram

You are asked to review an electrocardiogram (ECG) in the emergency department. Helpfully, a summary of details is printed at the top as follows: Rate 88/min, regular rhythm, axis –20°, PR duration 0.26 seconds (constant), QRS complex 0.08 seconds, QT interval 0.2 seconds. You note that P-waves are only present before each QRS and that the rhythm is regular.

Which of the following would be the best summary?

A First-degree heart block
B Left axis deviation
C Left bundle branch block
D Refuse to summarise until it can be compared with an old ECG
E Ventricular tachycardia

20. Investigation of deranged liver function tests

A 65-year-old man with a long-standing diagnosis of chronic obstructive pulmonary disease has been reviewed by his GP for deteriorating liver function tests and clinical signs and symptoms of cirrhosis. The patient reports his mother also having lung and liver pathology; however, he can't expand any further on this.

What investigation should the GP arrange?

A Alpha-1-antitrypsin serum levels
B Alpha-fetoprotein levels
C Anti–smooth muscle antibodies
D Gamma GT levels
E Hepatitis screen

21. Epigastric pain

A 44-year-old woman presents to the emergency department with pain. The pain is epigastric, sharp in nature, worse on lying flat and during inspiration. She has recently suffered a chest infection. She is not a smoker. On examination, she has diffuse inspiratory crepitations. Her oxygen saturation is 98% on room air. Her ECG shows widespread, saddle-shaped ST elevation.

Which of the following is the most likely diagnosis?

A Acute pericarditis
B Angina
C Myocardial infarction
D Pleurisy
E Pulmonary embolism

22. Gout prophylaxis

A 55-year-old overweight pub landlord presents with a several-year history of episodic acute painful joint swelling that started in his left big toe and now affects his knees. Symptoms improve with use of diclofenac. Gout was diagnosed on his first hospital visit; however, this now appears recurrent. He developed an acute attack in his left knee 2 days ago.

Which of the following represents the best plan for prophylaxis?

A Keep on long-term diclofenac with gastric protection
B Start allopurinol now with non-steroidal anti-inflammatory drug (NSAID) cover and increase until his urate is below 300 mmol/L
C Start allopurinol at least 2 weeks after the acute attack has settled with NSAID cover and increase until his urate level is below 300 mmol/L
D Switch to long-term colchicine
E Switch to use of depot steroid injections

23. Hepatomegaly

Which of the following conditions does not classically cause hepatomegaly?

A End-stage cirrhosis
B Fatty liver
C Hepatocellular carcinoma
D Myeloproliferative disease
E Right-sided heart failure

24. Sclerosing cholangitis

Which of the following conditions is associated with sclerosing cholangitis?

A Autoimmune hepatitis
B Coeliac disease
C Irritable bowel syndrome
D Pernicious anaemia
E Ulcerative colitis (UC)

25. Investigation of status epilepticus

A 35-year-old homeless man presents to the emergency department in a state of unconsciousness. He was fitting when the ambulance crew got to him 20 minutes ago, and a friend at the scene estimated that he had started fitting "around 15 minutes before". His friend informed the ambulance crew that he is a known epileptic, and you find a pack of phenytoin on him. He looks dishevelled and smells of alcohol. His blood pressure is 170/95 mmHg and temperature 37.9°C. On examination there is a quiet systolic murmur, though it is difficult to fully characterise.

Which of the following investigations will be most useful at this stage?

A Computed tomography (CT) of the brain
B Echocardiogram
C Electroencephalogram (EEG)
D Magnetic resonance imaging (MRI) of the brain
E Phenytoin levels

26. Shortness of breath

A 74-year-old male has a developing history over the last month of shortness of breath. He is coughing up frothy white sputum, which recently has contained a small amount of blood. On examination, his chest demonstrates diffuse crackles on inspiration through which you can just discern a mid-diastolic murmur and a loud first heart sound. His chest X-ray confirms pulmonary oedema.

What is the most likely underlying cause for his symptoms?

A Lower respiratory tract infection
B Mitral stenosis
C Non–small cell carcinoma of the lung
D Pulmonary embolism
E Small cell carcinoma of the lung

27. Aortic regurgitation

In clinic, a retired 62-year-old man presents with shortness of breath on exertion. You find a collapsing pulse and subsequent echocardiography confirms aortic regurgitation.

Which of the following is NOT associated with aortic regurgitation?

A Ankylosing spondylosis
B Aortic dissection
C Marfan syndrome
D Rheumatic fever
E Systemic lupus erythematosus (SLE)

28. Management of oliguria

A previously fit and well 70-year-old woman was admitted due to a fractured neck of the femur, and has recently returned to the ward after a cemented hemiarthroplasty. You are bleeped to see her, it is noted that she's had only 30 mL urine output in the last 3 hours. She is asleep, with a patient-controlled analgesic device in situ. Her airway is intact, and respiratory rate is 12/min with normal saturations and good air entry bilaterally. Her pulse is 125 bpm and blood pressure is 95/68 mmHg, and she has delayed capillary refill. She has pale conjunctiva and a temperature of 37.3°C. She has a 12-hourly bag of normal saline running. Her catheter is draining concentrated urine. An abdominal exam is normal.

Which of the following interventions would you try first to increase the urine output?

A Fluid challenge of 500 mL 5% dextrose over 10 minutes
B Fluid challenge of 500 mL normal saline over 10 minutes
C Flush the catheter
D Start antibiotics for presumed sepsis
E Stop the patient-controlled analgesic device

29. Steatorrhoea

A 23-year-old woman visits you about her stools, which over the last couple of months, have become extremely foul smelling, pale in colour and difficult to flush. This has been associated with vague abdominal pains and a bloating sensation. She finds this embarrassing, as she lives in a shared house. She is normally fit and well.

What is the most likely diagnosis?

A Chronic pancreatitis
B Coeliac disease
C Common bile duct obstruction
D Cystic fibrosis
E *Giardia* infection

30. Management of Parkinson's disease

An 83-year-old man who was diagnosed as having Parkinson's disease 3 years ago has been treated with levodopa (L-DOPA). Whilst he initially responded well to therapy, he has started to be increasingly still and has fallen more in the last 4 months despite no intercurrent illness or change in L-DOPA therapy.

Which is the best management option?

A Add a dopamine agonist (e.g. ropinirole)
B Add a peripheral dopamine antagonist (e.g. domperidone)
C Decrease L-DOPA therapy
D Increase L-DOPA therapy
E Stop L-DOPA therapy

31. Autoantibodies

Which antibody can you expect to see in primary biliary cirrhosis (PBC)?

A ANA
B ANCA
C Anti-mitochondrial antibody
D Antiphospholipid antibodies
E Anti–smooth muscle antibodies

32. Coronary circulation

The left anterior descending coronary artery usually supplies:

A The anterior wall of the left ventricle and the atrioventricular node
B The anterior wall of the left ventricle and the interventricular septum
C The anterior wall of the left ventricle, atrioventricular node and interventricular septum
D The interventricular septum and the inferior part of the left ventricle
E The sinoatrial node, the atrioventricular node and the inferior part of the left ventricle

33. Management of anaemia

A 42-year-old woman with menorrhagia is complaining of tiredness. The GP does some blood tests, which reveal hypochromic microcytic anaemia, a decreased ferritin level and a raised total iron binding capacity. Platelets were slightly raised.

Which of the following is the best treatment for this anaemia?

A Erythropoietin
B Iron chelators
C Iron supplementation
D Regular transfusion
E Regular venesection

34. ACE inhibitors

In which of the following circumstances should angiotensin-converting enzyme (ACE) inhibitors be avoided where possible?

A Glomerulonephritis
B Lupus nephritis
C Renal artery stenosis
D Systemic sclerosis with renal involvement
E All of the above

35. Microbiology

Which of the following correctly describes *Staphylococcus aureus*?

A Anaerobic rod
B Gram-negative coccus
C Gram-negative rod
D Gram-positive coccus
E Gram-positive rod

36. Skin lesions

A 78-year-old retired groundskeeper presents with a 2-cm skin lump on his temple. He is unsure how long it has been there. It appears to have a rolled, shiny edge with telangiectasia and a central ulcerated area.

Which of the following is the most likely diagnosis?

A Actinic keratosis
B Basal cell carcinoma
C Keratoacanthoma
D Malignant melanoma
E Squamous cell carcinoma

37. Diagnosis of abdominal pain

A 54-year-old woman presents to the emergency department with a 2-month history of intermittent right upper quadrant pain. The pain is sharp in nature and radiates round to the back. On examination there is no jaundice and no hepatomegaly, and she is apyrexial. Liver function tests and an amylase are normal. She has no history of recent foreign travel.

What is the most likely diagnosis?

A Biliary colic
B Cholangitis
C Hepatitis A
D Hepatitis C
E Pancreatitis

38. Ankylosing spondylitis

A 23-year-old man presents with a month-long history of lower back pain and stiffness.

Which of the following symptoms would make you think of ankylosing spondylitis (AS) as the diagnosis?

A Asymmetrical tenderness on palpation over the lumbosacral spine
B HLA-DR4 genotype
C Pain present on waking in the early morning
D Scoliosis present on examination
E Worse after heavy lifting

39. Mitral stenosis

A 75-year-old woman in the pre-assessment clinic tells you she has mitral stenosis.

Which of the following is NOT a sign of mitral stenosis?

A Bifid P-wave
B Diastolic opening snap heart sound
C Double impulse apex beat
D Mid-diastolic murmur
E Peripheral cyanosis

40. Management of facial weakness

A 35-year-old man presents with a 2-day history of right-sided facial weakness. He is otherwise fit and well. There is no past history of neurological symptoms or preceding infection. On examination, the middle ear is normal, the salivary glands are not enlarged, and no other cranial nerves are affected. The forehead is not spared. Neurological examination of the limbs is unremarkable. Routine investigations are all normal.

Which of the following represents the most appropriate management plan?

A Aspirin, dipyridamole, a statin and an angiotensin-converting enzyme (ACE) inhibitor
B Penicillin-based antibiotic therapy and antiviral therapy
C Steroids
D Steroids and penicillin-based antibiotic therapy
E Steroids, antiviral therapy and eye protection

41. Pathological fracture

A 51-year-old man is found to have a pathological fracture of his femur. Investigations reveal immunoglobulin light chains in the urine.

What is his diagnosis?

A Benign monoclonal gammopathy
B Bone metastases
C Multiple myeloma
D Osteoporosis
E Vitamin D deficiency

42. Management of HIV

A 35-year-old man is diagnosed with human immunodeficiency virus (HIV) infection.

Which of the following indicates that highly active antiretroviral therapy (HAART) should be commenced?

A All patients with HIV
B Viral load > 50 copies/mL
C Viral load > 100 copies/mL
D CD4 count < 200 cells/mm^3
E CD4 count < 500 cells/mm^3

43. Tetralogy of Fallot

An anxious mum has read on the internet about tetralogy of Fallot, as she is convinced her little boy may have it.

Which of the following is least likely to be associated with the diagnosis?

A Her child is small for his age
B Her child is cyanotic
C His pulse exhibits a radiofemoral delay
D Her child exhibits a loud systolic murmur
E Her child can relive his symptoms by squatting

44. Investigation of dysphagia

A 65-year-old man presents with intermittent difficulty in swallowing for the last 4 months. This is associated with regurgitation. He has not paid attention to his weight so cannot comment on weight loss but has felt tired recently and noticed his stool to be darker than normal. He smokes 20 cigarettes a day and has done so for the last 40 years. He does not drink alcohol. What is the most important investigation in this case?

A Barium swallow
B Chest X-ray
C CT of the chest
D Endoscopy
E Iron studies

45. Thalassaemia trait

A 55-year-old Asian man with known thalassaemia trait registers with a new GP and is found to have a mild microcytic anaemia on routine testing. He does not complain of any symptoms.

What is the most appropriate treatment?

A Blood transfusion
B Folate supplementation
C Iron chelators
D Iron supplementation
E No treatment required

46. Warfarin therapy

A 72-year-old man is on warfarin for atrial fibrillation. Following a recent chest infection, his international normalised ratio (INR) rockets up to 5.2.

What was the most likely cause for this?

A Codeine phosphate
B Erythromycin
C Inappropriate high doses of warfarin
D INR increased in concomitant infection
E Steroid inhalers

47. The painful joint

A 40-year-old man with a past history of a right knee replacement 2 years ago limps into the emergency department with an acutely red, hot, swollen and exquisitely tender right knee, which he holds rigid. His observations are stable.

Which of the following represents the best approach to diagnosis and management?

A Bloods including FBC, UE, CRP and urate, blood cultures, XR, aspirate knee followed by IV antibiotics
B Bloods including FBC, UE, CRP and urate, blood cultures, XR, IV antibiotics, discussion with registrar regarding washout in theatre
C Bloods including FBC, UE, CRP and urate, blood cultures, XR, discussion with registrar regarding washout in theatre
D Urgent transfer to theatre for washout
E Discharge home with oral antibiotics

48. The unresponsive patient

A 29-year-old man is brought to the emergency department having been found unresponsive on a park bench. On examination, his airway is patent and he has a spontaneous respiratory rate of 7, with a saturation rate of 92% on air. There is no abnormality on examination or auscultation of the chest. He has a pulse of 70 bpm and a blood pressure of 110/80 mmHg. The ECG is normal. He has a Glasgow Coma Score (GCS) of 9 and has pinpoint pupils. He has a temperature of 36.8°C and a blood sugar reading of 6. Basic initial management steps include high-flow oxygen administration and intravenous access.

Which of the following might you also implement?

A 500 mL stat intravenous fluid challenge
B 50 mL of 50% glucose intravenously stat
C Bair hugger
D Flumazenil
E Naloxone

49. Vomiting

A first-time mother comes to visit you with her 10-month-old son. At least once every day her son vomits up his entire feed. The vomiting is not projectile, but rather the feed returns to the mouth and spills over his top. She stopped breastfeeding him when he was 6 months old. He is otherwise well in himself, with a normal weight for his age.

What is the most likely diagnosis?

A Gastro-oesophageal reflux disease
B Lactose intolerance
C Physiological posseting
D Pyloric stenosis
E Viral gastroenteritis

50. Weight loss

A 13-year-old girl, who is quiet and withdrawn, comes to see you with her mother. She has a 4-month history of weight loss and secondary amenorrhoea. She has no bowel symptoms. Her body mass index (BMI) is 16 kg/m². Apart from being very thin, the examination is otherwise normal. All blood results, including hormone assays, are normal.

What is the most likely diagnosis?

A Anorexia nervosa
B Coeliac disease
C Crohn's disease
D Epstein–Barr virus infection
E Irritable bowel syndrome

Practice paper 1: Answers

1. Acute coronary syndrome (ACS)

B. Give 75 mg aspirin stat

A stat dose of 300 mg aspirin is the correct figure. Low-dose (75 mg) aspirin is used for long-term prevention. ACS is the name given to a collection of cardiac diseases that all share the same atherosclerotic aetiology. ST-elevated myocardial infarction (MI), non-ST-elevated MI and unstable angina are all caused by stenosed coronary arteries starving the myocardium of oxygen (angina), leading to hypoxic cell death (MI). Unstable angina occurs on the cusp of these phenomena, when a rest is no longer adequate to replenish the myocardium with oxygen. ACSs are usually caused by intimal plaque rupture leading to an intraluminal thrombus. Aspirin, clopidogrel and heparin aim to prevent platelets binding and therefore to arrest thrombus growth and dissolve the thrombus. Aspirin can cause stomach ulcers, and so, in order to balance risks and benefits, low-dose aspirin is given long term; a higher dose (300 mg) is given acutely. Statins lower serum cholesterol, and their use is thought to reduce plaque formation. ACE inhibitors and beta-blockers reduce afterload and heart rate, lowering the heart's oxygen demand and thus reducing the risk of further ischaemic events.

2. Obstructive renal impairment

E. Systemic sclerosis

Benign prostatic hyperplasia is seen in 40% of men over the age of 60. It is caused by a proliferation of the central transitional zone of the prostate. It typically presents with poor flow, dribbling and nocturia but may also lead to urine infections, stones and acute or chronic retention with overflow incontinence. Management is varied and includes lifestyle changes, medication including tamsulosin and finasteride or surgical removal, either via the urethra (minimally invasive) or in an open manner. The sequelae of the pathology needs to be weighed against the potential complications of treatment, including a 15% risk of impotence associated with transurethral resection of the prostate.

DOI: 10.1201/9781003648222-2

Recurrent kidney stones passing into the ureter can cause scarring, especially at narrow sites such as the vesicoureteric junction.

Retroperitoneal fibrosis typically involves an autoimmune fibrosing inflammatory reaction starting in the vasa vasorum of the aorta and spreading throughout the retroperitoneum. It is typically seen in smokers and those with other autoimmune conditions such as systemic lupus erythematosus (SLE). The ureters can become embedded within the fibrous tissue, thus leading to bilateral hydronephrosis and the need for retrograde stent insertion/ureterolysis.

Schistosomiasis is caused by a parasite common in the Middle East and parts of Africa. It may cause obstructive renal impairment via the eggs directly blocking the ureter or via the formation of a bladder tumour.

Systemic sclerosis is an autoimmune condition that has the potential to involve multiple organs including skin, lungs and heart. CREST syndrome is a form of limited systemic sclerosis. Systemic sclerosis can lead to renal failure; however, this is due to a reduction of renal perfusion secondary to afferent arteriole sclerosis as opposed to an obstructive uropathy.

3. Management of skin lesions

C. Excisional biopsy

This lesion is 8 mm in size, growing, with a keratotic horn and has bled. These are concerning features of a skin cancer. It is in a sun exposed site and thus a squamous cell carcinoma cannot be ruled out without a pathological diagnosis. Using a suitable margin the area should be excised and closed directly or may require a full-thickness skin graft or local flap coverage. The other options do not give a pathological diagnosis.

4. Chest X-ray

A. Trachea deviated to the right, dull to percussion of RUZ, reduced breath sounds on auscultation

In bronchogenic carcinoma, lobar collapse is likely secondary to bronchi obstruction from the malignancy. It can, however, also be seen in foreign body aspiration or mucus plug.

A lung collapse would tend to pull the trachea towards the affected side. There would be reduced breath sounds (with or without crackles and bronchial breathing) and dullness to percussion on the affected side.

5. Headaches

D. Polycythaemia rubra vera

Myeloproliferative disorders occur following proliferation of myeloid stem cells. Such conditions may be primary, such as polycythaemia vera (PCV), or secondary following COPD, synthetic erythropoietin (EPO) administration or EPO-secreting malignancies.

Polycythaemia rubra vera is a myeloproliferative disorder characterised by a raised haemoglobin level, red cell count and packed cell volume (haematocrit). *JAK2* mutations are seen in 90% of cases. As a result, the blood becomes extremely viscous, causing an increased risk of arterial and venous thrombosis and paradoxical bleeding. Patients often complain of headaches, visual disturbance, lethargy and pruritus that is classically worse after bathing in warm water. Signs include facial plethora, splenomegaly and gout. Investigations include full blood count and bone marrow biopsy. Treatment of the polycythaemia rubra vera involves either venesection (blood-letting) or chemotherapy (hydroxyurea) with prophylactic aspirin, with an aim of keeping haematocrit below 0.45. If treated appropriately patients tend to survive for many years and often die from non-related causes. Approximately 30% of patients will develop myelofibrosis, and 5% will develop acute myeloid leukaemia as part of the disease's natural history.

6. Chronic obstructive pulmonary disease

C. Add in long-acting beta-agonist (salmeterol) with long-acting muscarinic antagonist (tiotropium)

COPD is irreversible and is characterised by chronic bronchitis and emphysema. Patients commonly have a history of smoking, and they suffer from breathlessness, cough, chronic sputum production, wheeze and reduced exercise tolerance. Typically, patients progress in terms of severity and have frequent exacerbations, especially during the winter. They are at high risk of pneumothorax and lung cancer. It is diagnosed from pulmonary function tests of FEV_1 <80% and FEV_1/FVC ratio <0.7. Management starts with educating the patient on their condition, smoking cessation, healthy diet/exercise and annual vaccinations, as well as formal pulmonary rehabilitation programmes. This is supplemented with short-acting PRN inhalers in the form of beta-agonists (salbutamol) or antimuscarinics (ipratropium). In this gentleman, despite using PRN salbutamol, he feels his breathing is progressively worse. As a result, after ensuring effective inhaler technique, the addition of a long-acting beta-agonist with a long-acting muscarinic antagonist (tiotropium), as he has no asthmatic features, is the next step. He does not need admission, as he is clinically stable. He should be advised to attend the accident and emergency department if he does become acutely unwell.

7. Management of asthma

D. Leukotriene receptor antagonists

The altered level of consciousness, exhaustion, silent chest, PaO_2 <8.0 kPa and "normal $PaCO_2$" 4.6–6.0 kPa all suggest that this patient has life-threatening asthma. High-flow oxygen is needed to maintain a saturation level of 94–98%. In acute life-threatening asthma, the nebulised route (oxygen driven) is recommended. Steroids reduce mortality, relapses, subsequent hospital admission and requirement for beta-2 agonist therapy. Magnesium sulphate has bronchodilation effects and is used in acute severe asthma if there is not a good initial response to inhaled bronchodilator therapy and also in life-threatening asthma. There is insufficient evidence at present to show that leukotriene receptor antagonists are effective in the management of acute asthma. Be aware that the altered level of consciousness may also be due to a rising CO_2, which is an indication of near-fatal asthma, thus requiring intensive care unit (ICU) referral and ventilatory support. Critical care should be involved at the earliest recognition of deterioration.

8. Collapse

E. Hypoglycaemia

When assessing a patient with collapse, it is essential to establish whether it was syncope (loss of consciousness) or non-syncope. Common causes of syncope include vasovagal, arrhythmia or cardiac structural abnormality, postural hypotension and carotid insufficiency. Non-syncopal causes include seizures and hypoglycaemia.

This patient has no risk factors for carotid artery stenosis.

Hypertrophic obstructive cardiomyopathy (HOCM) is a congenital disease of the myocardium. The left ventricular myocardium becomes so thick that the outflow tract becomes restricted. This restriction is mechanically exacerbated by the muscular systolic contraction generated by vigorous exercise; hence, hard exercise leads to a fall-off in output, which leads to syncope. Sufferers are vulnerable to sudden death, of which there may be a family history, as the disease is inherited (autosomal dominant).

There is no indication this was an epileptic seizure, especially as there was no reported jerking, tongue biting or incontinence.

Vasovagal episodes are the most common cause of syncope; however, this patient's history points towards hypoglycaemia. He had a binge of alcohol the night before, poor sleep and then strenuous exercise. He is also demonstrating signs of a sympathetic response and agitation secondary to the reduced sugar levels. You check his blood sugar, and a reading of 2.5 mmol/L prompts you to treat with oral glucose solution and a starch-based meal. If he had reduced consciousness, you could use either IV dextrose or IM glucagon. He should be investigated for potential first presentation of diabetes mellitus.

9. Eczema versus psoriasis

C. Localised to flexures rather than extensors

Nail changes are much more commonly associated with psoriasis, usually with nail pitting and onycholysis (detachment of parts of the nail from the nail bed) and occasionally with subungual hyperkeratosis (extensive keratotic growth beneath the nail). Distal interphalangeal joint disease (in this case with pain and swelling) is one of five characteristic patterns of "psoriatic arthropathy", which overall around 5–10% of those with psoriasis will develop at some stage – in some cases, before the outbreak of psoriasis. The five patterns are distal interphalangeal arthritis, symmetrical polyarthritis, asymmetrical oligoarthritis, spondyloarthropathy and arthritis mutilans, which is a severe destructive arthropathy mainly affecting the hands. X-rays of the distal joints of the hand may show destructive erosive changes progressing to a "pencil in cup" sign. Eczema is more commonly localised to flexures, whereas psoriatic plaques are more typically localised to extensor surfaces. Psoriasis more often presents with well-demarcated lesions, or "plaques", whereas eczematous lesions more often are described as "patches" and are more diffuse. Psoriatic plaques can occur following trauma, called the "Koebner effect".

10. Diagnosis of multiple sclerosis

D. Periventricular white matter lesions not necessarily matching the clinical picture

Longitudinally extensive transverse myelitis is unusual in multiple sclerosis (MS) and is more typical of neuromyelitis optica (NMO or Devic's disease), a rare autoimmune central nervous system (CNS) demyelinating disease affecting the spinal cord and optic nerves. Once thought to be a subtype of MS, it is now known to be a distinct disease strongly associated with anti-aquaporin-4 antibodies. Whilst grey matter is affected in MS, and there is some evidence that overall grey matter volume decreases in MS and correlates with disability, focal grey matter inflammatory lesions would not be expected, and the focal lesions are in fact found in the white matter. The cerebellum and brainstem are affected in MS, although not exclusively. White matter lesions are classically described as "periventricular", and the lesions found do not always correlate with a clinical focus of disease. This is because the CNS inflammation does not always cause demyelination or axonal damage of clinical significance, and the CNS can recover from these foci of inflammation.

11. The multidisciplinary team

A. District nurse

District nurses provide care within the community. Their workload includes looking after house-bound and recently discharged patients, helping them manage wound dressings and administering medications, stoma and catheter care. Their role is fundamental to ease transition into community care, thus reducing hospital stay. Reducing hospital stay not only minimises the risk of hospital-acquired infections but also frees up beds and is cost-effective for the National Health Service (NHS). Emphasising the importance of community services, the new NHS long-term plan has allocated a further £4.5 billion to such services.

Social workers look after the individuals and their contacts from a social perspective (e.g. families, friends). They also liaise with other organisations, including schools, the NHS, housing agencies and charitable organisations, to plan packages of care and support for the individual. The health visitor (a qualified nurse) takes over care of a newborn from community midwives after the first 10 days of birth. Health visitors also run health promotion and smoking cessation clinics. An orthotist is someone who measures, designs and fits orthoses (an external device that can be applied to correct a deformity, rather like a splint).

Orthotics, from Greek *ortho* = straighten

12. Diagnosis of chest pain

B. CXR

This young gentleman is complaining of post-operative pleuritic chest pain following clavicle fracture fixation. Although both an ECG and blood tests are useful to explore other potential differentials for chest pain, including pulmonary embolism and chest infection, based on this history, a diagnosis of left-sided pneumothorax is most likely, and thus CXR is the most useful test. One of the risks of clavicle fixation is pneumothorax, and this must be discussed with the patient pre-operatively. A trauma CT is not appropriate in this setting, and intraoperative images are not likely to show the full chest and may not show an established pneumothorax caused iatrogenically.

13. Risk factors for ischaemic heart disease

E. Consuming 12 units of alcohol a week

According to the American Heart Association, moderate alcohol consumption can reduce coronary artery disease. In the UK, the recommended allowance is 14 units of alcohol per week for both men and women (ideally spread over 3 or more days with several alcohol-free days during the week too). Raised high-density lipoprotein (HDL) and reducing clotting potential helps to reduce risk. All the other options increase the risk of ischaemic heart disease.

14. Diagnosis of cough

C. *Legionella pneumophila*

L. pneumophila tends to colonise in water tanks kept at below 60°C (e.g. hotel air-conditioning and hot water systems). Patients who acquire *L. pneumophila* infection will present with non-specific symptoms such as fever, myalgia, headache, confusion and diarrhoea. Blood tests reveal hyponatraemia and abnormal liver function tests (elevated liver enzymes, hypoalbuminaemia). The diagnosis is confirmed by *Legionella* serology or urine *Legionella* antigen.

15. Diagnosis of vertigo

B. Delayed onset (a few seconds) torsional nystagmus on descent facing one side only

Benign paroxysmal positional vertigo (BPPV) is caused by debris blocking the normal flow of endolymph in the labyrinth, leading to misreporting of positional change by the vestibules and a discrepancy between actual position and the position of the head according to the vestibules. Thus, nystagmus occurs as two different inputs compete for different oculomotor outputs, and vertigo (the perception that the world is moving) ensues. This happens only when the head moves; there is no vertigo with a still head. It usually affects one side only, and thus Hallpike's manoeuvre (described next) only reveals nystagmus when the patient's head is tilted back whilst they face one side and not the other. Torsional nystagmus is normally seen after a few seconds of the head being tilted back – it is important to keep the patient lying back for some time. The nystagmus should wear off after around 20 seconds, and on repeat testing it lasts a shorter amount of time ("fatiguing"). This is the basis of vestibular exercises, which are designed so that compensatory mechanisms may be induced more swiftly, and the vertigo attacks will thus become less frequent and less disabling.

The Hallpike test is conducted as follows:

1. The patient sits upright with their legs extended.
2. The patient's head is then rotated to one side at a 45-degree angle.
3. The patient is then made to lie down quickly, and the head is held in extension (should hang slightly over the edge of the bed).
4. The patient's eyes are then observed. A positive test will result in nystagmus towards the affected side after a 5- to 10-second latent period.

The Epley manoeuvre effectively treats most cases of BPPV. In this manoeuvre:

1. The patient sits upright with their legs extended.
2. The patient's head is rotated 45 degrees toward the affected ear.
3. The patient is quickly laid back so that the head is hanging off the edge of the couch slightly (as in the Hallpike position) and held for 30 seconds.
4. The patient's head is then turned 90 degrees toward the opposite side (without lifting) and held for 30 seconds.
5. The patient is rolled onto their side (so the face is almost facing the floor) and held for 30 seconds.
6. The patient is slowly helped up into a sitting position while keeping the head slightly flexed and turned and held for 30 seconds.
7. The patient's head is turned back to the midline with the neck flexed 45 degrees (for 30 seconds).

Charles Skinner Hallpike, English otologist (1900-1979)

16. Epistaxis

E. Granulomatosis with polyangiitis

Granulomatosis with polyangiitis (GPA, formally known as Wegener granulomatosis) is characterised by systemic vasculitis that involves small and medium vessels. The classic triad consists of upper and lower respiratory tract involvement and pauci-immune glomerulonephritis. The upper respiratory tract involvement includes otorrhoea, sinusitis, nasal discharge and crusting, epistaxis, oral and nasal ulcers, mucosal bleeding and inflammation, nasal septal perforation and a saddle nose deformity. The lower respiratory tract involvement includes cough, haemoptysis, chest pain and shortness of breath. Microscopic haematuria is a common finding in GPA. A positive antineutrophil cytoplasmic antibody (ANCA) test in the setting of this classic triad is sufficient to diagnose GPA without a histological confirmation. Goodpasture syndrome is caused by an anti–glomerular basement membrane antibody that results in pulmonary haemorrhage and glomerulonephritis without involvement of the upper respiratory tract.

Friedrich Wegener, German pathologist (1907-1990)

17. Diarrhoea

B. *Clostridium difficile* infection

C. difficile is a major cause of antibiotic-associated diarrhoea and hospital morbidity within the UK. *C. difficile* is a Gram-positive commensal bacterium of the gastrointestinal tract that can proliferate when the intestinal flora is disturbed by the use of broad-spectrum antibiotics. Third-generation cephalosporins clindamycin and fluoroquinolones are particularly implicated with this. Elderly individuals and those with underlying health conditions are at higher risk, and the prescription of such antibiotics should be undertaken with great care and consideration of risk versus benefit to the individual patient. *C. difficile* produces two enterotoxins (A and B) that cause severe inflammation of the intestinal mucosa and the formation of thick fibrous bands (pseudo-membranes, i.e. fibrinopurulent exudates that consist of inflammatory cells, fibrin, and necrotic tissue) in the intestine, which can harbour large numbers of bacteria. The patient often has significant diarrhoea (with or without blood), which can lead to rapid dehydration, electrolyte imbalance and death. *C. difficile* is treated by managing the patient's fluid and electrolyte balance and prescribing a course of metronidazole or vancomycin. Much effort is being placed in the prevention of *Clostridium* infection by promoting the correct use of broad-spectrum antibiotics and educating staff and visitors regarding the importance of hand washing. It should be noted that the spores of *C. difficile* are not destroyed by alcohol hand gel, meaning that soap and water must be used every time! Although *C. difficile* is the most likely diagnosis, the patient's stool sample should be sent for analysis with the patient placed in isolation. One should liaise with trust policy, as infectious disease and public health departments may need notifying. Adenocarcinoma of the gastrointestinal tract can present with altered bowel motions – "common things are common" – and we have a more likely infectious cause in this case.

Clostridium, from Latin *kloster* = spindle (shape)

Difficile, from Latin *difficile* = difficult

18. Diagnosis of malaria

E. Three thick and thin blood films on consecutive days

Falciparum antigen dipstick testing is a useful, cheap and a low-effort method for diagnosing or excluding *falciparum* malaria; however, a well-examined blood film is far more sensitive. Thick and thin blood films are done because thick films make pickup of low-level parasitaemias more likely, and thin blood films allow species identification and quantification (more than 2% of red blood cells being parasitised is a prognostic marker of severe disease). Blood films should be taken on 3 consecutive days, as an initial film may be negative due to the lifecycle of the parasite. Blood cultures should be taken, as there may be coexisting bacteraemia ("algid malaria"); however, they do not grow *Plasmodium* species. Liver biopsy is not used to investigate malaria.

19. Electrocardiogram

A. First-degree heart block

Analyse an ECG methodically. Start with rate: bradycardia if less than 60/min, tachycardia if greater than 100/min. Next, check the rhythm is regular;

this can be trickier than it seems, especially if the patient is tachycardic. The axis is determined by looking at the amplitude of the QRS complex relative to lead II, i.e. lead II is 0°, lead I is −45° and lead III is +135°. If the QRS amplitude is greatest in lead II and leads I and III have identical, lesser magnitudes, then the QRS is not deviated. If it is most positive in lead I, then it is deviated to the left. If it is most positive in lead III, then it is deviated to the right. Remember that the QRS complex is the charge "washing" through the myocardium. The axis of the QRS helps us to visualise the comparative muscularity of the right and left ventricles, which may in turn highlight a disease process against which a given ventricle is fighting, e.g. aortic stenosis leading to left ventricular hypertrophy resulting in left axis deviation. An axis outside of ±30 degrees can be said to be deviated. The P-wave position and shape should be noted. The PR interval should be less than 0.20 seconds. In this case, there is a fixed delay (through the atrioventricular node), which is called first-degree heart block. Second-degree heart block can have both a Wenckebach pattern, where there is an increasing PR interval before loss of a QRS complex, and a fixed 2: or 3:1 ratio between P-waves and QRS complexes. Third-degree or complete heart block has complete dislocation between P-waves and QRS. Once the PR interval has been assessed, one should examine the QRS amplitude, shape and duration, which are all significant. A width >3 small squares (at 25 mm/s ECG speed) is equivalent to 0.12 seconds, and this is the boundary between QRS complexes being narrow or broad. Ventricular tachycardias are broad (and faster than 90/min). A broad complex may well contain a distortion in shape in one of the leads, indicating bundle branch block. This ECG has a narrow QRS complex. One should assess the ST segment for signs of ischaemia. Finally, the T-wave size and the QT duration should be observed. It is always good practice to compare a current ECG to a previous ECG, but this should not prevent you reviewing and summarising the ECG. If there is any doubt and no old ECGs are available, a repeat test can be requested to look for dynamic changes. As a general rule, one should always correlate the ECG findings with the clinical picture.

20. Investigation of deranged liver function tests

A. Alpha-1-antitrypsin serum levels

When investigating such patients, all the listed tests should be explored; however, with a significant family and personal history of both COPD and liver disease, alpha-1-antitrypsin (A1AT) deficiency should be the first to be considered. A1AT deficiency is an autosomal recessive disorder. Approximately 1% of COPD patients will have this genetic abnormality. A1AT is a serine protease inhibitor normally synthesised in the liver whose role is to cleave and inhibit the proteolytic enzyme neutrophil elastase. Absence of A1AT leads to pulmonary emphysema and liver disease in some patients.

The gene is located on chromosome 14, and there are variants that correlate to disease severity and presentation. The most severe forms can present with cirrhosis in childhood. Treatment is supportive.

Be aware that although A1AT should be investigated in this patient with a strong family history, one should not neglect common causes of liver disease, including alcohol consumption and gamma GT levels.

Smooth muscle antibodies are seen in autoimmune hepatitis. Alpha-fetoprotein is often raised in hepatocellular carcinoma.

21. Epigastric pain

A. Acute pericarditis

The ECG shows widespread, saddle-shaped ST elevation, a typical change associated with acute pericarditis. Pericarditis, although having many potential causes, is often caused by a preceding viral respiratory tract infection. It may also follow blunt trauma, radiotherapy or antiepileptic medication. This is a typical patient presentation, particularly the postural nature of the pain. Treatment is normally supportive with monotherapy or a combination of NSAIDs, aspirin and colchicine with associated proton pump inhibitor (PPI) cover. The patient should be monitored and advised to return promptly if symptoms worsen, as acute tamponade may occur due to the accumulation of inflammatory fluid in pericardium. Pleurisy (inflammation of the pleura) does not directly cause ECG changes and does not correlate as well with the sign of postural pain changes. Myocardial infarction and angina are unlikely to cause pain of this nature. A pulmonary embolism may have a similar presentation but may also affect the oxygen saturations. If ECG changes were present, they would not be saddle-shaped ST elevation, but rather sinus tachycardia (most common), S1Q3T3 (most classically associated) or others including right axis deviation and right bundle branch block (RBBB). Although unlikely, one must consider an arterial blood gas (ABG), as well as calculating the patient's Wells score.

22. Gout prophylaxis

C. Start allopurinol at least 2 weeks after the acute attack has settled with NSAID cover and increase until his urate level is below 300 mmol/L

Long-term use of diclofenac can lead to peptic ulceration and renal impairment and will achieve nothing between attacks, as there is no inflammation. Similarly, depot steroid injections may be used in acute attacks, but long-term steroids carry the risk of immunosuppression, as well as many other side effects. The underlying pathology in gout is hyperuricaemia; therefore, prophylactic treatment should aim to reduce serum urate. Allopurinol inhibits xanthine oxidase, which produces urate and thus lowers serum urate. It can precipitate acute attacks and therefore should not be used within 2–4 weeks of an acute attack and should be started with either NSAIDs or colchicine used at least 2 weeks before and 4 weeks after starting. Long-term colchicine is not recommended for prophylaxis. Sulfinpyrazone is a second-line prophylactic agent. Febuxostat, also an xanthine oxidase inhibitor, is generally recommended for those who are unable to take allopurinol due to adverse events or who have a poor response to allopurinol.

23. Hepatomegaly

A. End-stage cirrhosis

Hepatomegaly describes the enlargement of the liver. It is detected clinically by palpating the right upper quadrant during inspiration. As the patient inspires, the liver is displaced inferiorly by the lungs onto the examiner's hand. In normal individuals, the liver should not be palpated, with the exception of children and particularly thin patients. The presence of hepatomegaly is usually described in terms of size, e.g. number of fingerbreadths below the costal margin. The texture of the liver edge should also be documented, and it should be noted whether it is smooth or craggy. Conditions that cause hepatomegaly with a smooth margin include viral hepatitis, biliary tract obstruction, hepatic vein thrombosis (Budd–Chiari syndrome), right heart failure, alcohol excess and myeloproliferative disease. Hepatomegaly with a craggy border is usually associated with hepatic metastatic disease and polycystic disease.

End-stage cirrhosis does not result in hepatomegaly. Early liver damage often causes hepatomegaly and fatty infiltration, but as the damage progresses and fibrosis ensues, replacing the normal tissue architecture, the liver becomes small and scarred.

24. Sclerosing cholangitis

E. Ulcerative colitis (UC)

Sclerosing cholangitis is a condition causing inflammation, fibrosis and subsequent stricture formation of the bile ducts, leading to cholestasis and eventual cirrhosis. These changes occur in the intra- and extrahepatic bile ducts. There is a strong association with inflammatory bowel disease, most commonly UC, with about 80% of patients with sclerosing cholangitis having coexistent disease (note, though, that only ~5% of patients with UC have concomitant sclerosing cholangitis). These patients present with the effects of obstructive jaundice, which may include pruritus, yellow sclera, dark urine and pale faeces. Magnetic resonance cholangiopancreatography (MRCP) and liver function tests (LFTs) are used to make the diagnosis, with liver biopsies reserved for cases with diagnostic uncertainty. Liver biopsy characteristically demonstrates "onion skin" fibrosis around bile ducts, bile duct loss and fibrous scars. Treatment is primarily symptomatic;

ursodeoxycholic acid may delay disease progression, and cholestyramine is given to aid pruritus. Antibiotics +/– endoscopic retrograde cholangio-pancreatography (ERCP) are used if there is an acute bout of ascending cholangitis. Liver transplant is curative in some cases. Primary sclerosing cholangitis (PSC) also increases the risk of hepatic, bowel, pancreatic and gallbladder malignancy, and thus screening high-risk patients is recommended.

25. Investigation of status epilepticus

E. Phenytoin levels

There are many reasons why this man may be in status epilepticus, but the most common cause, and a quick and simple one to rule out, would be low antiepileptic drug levels. This is estimated to be the cause of around 30% of status epilepticus episodes. Alcoholism is prevalent amongst the homeless population, and many antiepileptics are metabolised by the cytochrome p450 system in the liver (phenytoin included). Chronic alcohol abuse can induce increased cytochrome p450 activity, which could then lower the phenytoin levels. His compliance with phenytoin therapy could be poor given his social situation. One should also remember alcohol withdrawal as a potential cause. Regarding the other investigations, brain imaging will be poor or impossible, as he is still fitting, and EEG is only indicated if he is still fitting after various management steps have been undertaken and he is taken to the intensive treatment unit (ITU) for general anaesthesia. Regarding the echocardiogram, the homeless population is indeed at risk of endocarditis, which could lead to subsequent septic embolisation to the brain, causing the seizures. A murmur is also heard; however, this would be a less likely cause than low phenytoin levels and less easy to treat acutely if found. Magnetic resonance imaging (MRI) of the head should be carried out beforehand if an intracranial cause such as septic emboli is being considered. Furthermore, regarding the possibly new murmur and fever, the fever could be due to the seizure activity, and the murmur could be benign or old (it may be worth contacting the GP or searching for the patient's old hospital notes to see if it has been investigated). One other important test to consider is blood glucose, as hypoglycaemia can be a simple reversible cause of status epilepticus.

26. Shortness of breath

B. Mitral stenosis

A history of recurrent rheumatic fever would reinforce this diagnosis. This patient's mitral valve is restricting the onward flow of freshly oxygenated blood from the lungs. This back pressure is the cause of his pulmonary oedema (inspiratory crackles and frothy sputum). The loud first heart sound is due to the mitral valve leaflets shutting abruptly at the start of systole, as if a door left ajar were closed with the same force as a door wide open. This can result from a stiffened mitral valve (commonly seen in mitral stenosis), which prevents the normal, gradual closure of the valve. The mid-diastolic murmur is the turbulent flow of blood through this restricted opening. It is low-frequency and so is best heard with the bell of the stethoscope. A malar flush may be visible upon the face of the patient.

Rheumatic fever is predominantly a disease of the developing world and is usually seen in children between 5 and 15 years of age. The condition develops 2–4 weeks after a group A beta-haemolytic streptococcal pharyngitis. In susceptible individuals, the antibodies formed against the bacterial carbohydrate cell wall cross-react with antigens in the heart, joints and skin in a process known as molecular mimicry. The immune response in the heart causes myocarditis, pericarditis and endocarditis, resulting in valve destruction, conduction defects, arrhythmia and congestive cardiac failure.

The diagnosis of rheumatic fever is made using the modified Duckett Jones criteria, requiring either two major criteria *or* one major and two minor criteria *plus* evidence of streptococcal infection (e.g. anti–streptolysin-O titres):

Modified Duckett Jones criteria

Major
- Pancarditis
- Polyarthritis
- Sydenham chorea (St Vitus's dance)
- Erythema marginatum
- Subcutaneous nodules

Minor
- Fever
- Arthralgia
- High erythrocyte sedimentation rate or white cell count
- Heart block

Chorea, from Latin *chorea* = dance

Saint Vitus's dance (*chorea sancti viti* in Latin) was a mediaeval festival that celebrated Vitus, the patron saint of dancers, actors and comedians

T Duckett Jones, American physician (1899-1954)

27. Aortic regurgitation

E. Systemic lupus erythematosus (SLE)

SLE can cause myocarditis, pericarditis and endocarditis. Whilst the latter manifestation can cause valvular vegetations, they are rarely symptomatic and are more likely to be diagnosed postmortem. Causes of aortic regurgitation, which presents primarily as dyspnoea, include idiopathic aortic root dilatation, syphilitic aortitis, aortic dissection and rheumatic fever. It is also associated with ankylosing spondylosis and Marfan syndrome. In addition to a collapsing pulse, aortic regurgitation also presents with an early diastolic murmur, a mid-diastolic rumble (Austin Flint murmur), de Musset's sign (synchronous head nodding), Quincke's sign (pulsing nail bed), Traube's sign ("pistol shot" sound over the femoral as the arterial walls snap taut due to the increased systolic pressure) and a laterally displaced apex beat.

Austin Flint, American physician (1812-1886)

Alfred de Musset, French novelist who died from aortic regurgitation. His brother noticed his head used to bob with his pulse

Heinrich Irenaeus Quincke, German physician (1842-1922)

Ludwig Traube, German physician (1818-1876)

28. Management of oliguria

B. Fluid challenge of 500 mL normal saline over 10 minutes

The normal urine output for an adult is 0.5 mL/kg/hr. Any post-operative patient who is hypotensive and tachycardia with poor urine output should be urgently assessed for causes of shock. The most likely diagnosis in this patient is post-operative hypovolaemia either from intraoperative blood loss and inadequate fluid replacement or a new reactive bleed. A reactive bleed occurs if a ligature slips or blood pressure increases post-operatively. The operation notes could be checked to confirm this. She is clinically dry with tachycardia, hypotension and delayed capillary refill and is thus showing signs of stage three hypovolaemic shock. Although a low-grade pyrexia is common post-operatively due to tissue damage, one must also consider sepsis as a potential diagnosis. In the immediate post-operative phase, however, hypovolaemic shock is a more likely diagnosis. This patient should be assessed in accident and emergency with high-flow O_2 provided before resuscitation fluids are administered. She does not have heart failure and should be able to tolerate a fluid challenge before reassessing hydration status. Normal saline should be used rather than 5% dextrose, as the saline will remain largely intravascular, whereas the 5% dextrose, after rapid metabolism of the dextrose, is essentially water, and this will enter the tissues and not increase the intravascular volume as much. It would be worth calling the transfusion department and ordering a couple of units of crossmatched blood. One should also examine the operative site, and the registrar should be informed in case the patient needs to return to theatre for haemostasis. Flushing the catheter can rule out obstruction of the catheter, but the bladder was not palpable on examination. Morphine does not commonly reduce urine output or lead to renal failure. It can cause urinary retention; however, a catheter is in situ so this is not the cause here.

29. Steatorrhoea

B. Coeliac disease

The description of this woman's stools is classical for steatorrhoea, which is a malabsorption of fat from the diet. There are many causes for this, including all of the above. However, coeliac disease is the most likely diagnosis in a woman of this age group with no other symptoms of respiratory distress or foreign travel. If the diagnosis is in doubt, repeated stool specimens should be sent for *Giardia* cysts and ova identification.

30. Management of Parkinson's disease

A. Add a dopamine agonist (e.g. ropinirole)

The general theory of Parkinson's disease management is that early on, when there are still many substantia nigra pars compacta (SNpc) neurones surviving, L-DOPA is more useful, as this precursor then increases the amount of dopamine being released in a physiological manner to allow movement. However, as the disease progresses and the SNpc neurones reduce in number, L-DOPA will not be able to increase the functional amount of dopamine being released in the basal ganglia, and so dopamine agonists are increasingly used. Dopamine agonists directly stimulate dopamine receptors in the basal ganglia, helping with movement control. Whilst they are less physiological than L-DOPA, they can still provide significant symptomatic relief, particularly for bradykinesia and postural instability. At the latter stage, increasing L-DOPA is unlikely to provide a benefit and may even contribute to dyskinesias; decreasing L-DOPA may be advisable but not without a dopamine agonist on board. Stopping L-DOPA entirely is likely to worsen function. The addition of a dopamine agonist at this stage, however, may relieve bradykinesia and postural instability but may also lead to hallucinations and compulsive behaviour. A peripheral dopamine antagonist (1) will not act centrally and (2) would exacerbate symptoms and so would be no help. Domperidone can in fact be used to relieve medication-associated nausea in Parkinson's disease.

31. Autoantibodies

C. Anti-mitochondrial antibody

Primary biliary cirrhosis (PBC), also known as primary biliary cholangitis, is a rare condition predominantly affecting women in their 50s. The aetiology is thought to be autoimmune. There is chronic granulomatous inflammation of the interlobular bile ducts causing cholestasis. Presentation is through the effects of cholestasis – jaundice, pruritus, hepatomegaly and pain. It may also be picked up early by deranged liver function tests in the asymptomatic patient. Diagnosis is confirmed by liver biopsy, and anti-mitochondrial antibodies (AMAs) may be present. Management is threefold: (1) symptomatic to reduce itchiness and prevent osteoporosis, (2) specific medications to improve absorption and (3) disease-modifying drugs such as ursodeoxycholic acid (which reduces cholestasis). Recent evidence, however, suggests that ursodeoxycholic acid does not improve mortality. Liver transplant may be an option in some candidates with end-stage disease.

32. Coronary circulation

B. The anterior wall of the left ventricle and the interventricular septum

The left anterior descending artery normally supplies the anterior wall of the left ventricle and the interventricular septum. It arises from the left coronary artery, as does the circumflex artery, which supplies the posterior and lateral sides of the left ventricle. The right coronary artery usually supplies the sinoatrial node, atrioventricular node, right ventricle and inferior part of the left ventricle. One should consider the coronary circulation when assessing an ECG with left anterior descending represented by V1–4, circumflex by V5, 6, 1 and aVL; and right coronary artery represented by II, III and aVF. A posterior myocardial infarction (MI) is usually caused by thrombosis to the posterior descending artery, which is a branch of the right coronary artery.

33. Management of anaemia

C. Iron supplementation

These blood tests reveal iron-deficiency anaemia (IDA), which is most commonly treated with oral iron supplementation.

IDA is defined as a haemoglobin concentration below 13.5 g/dL in males or 11.5 g/dL in females, in association with a low mean cell volume (MCV) and evidence of depleted iron stores (i.e. a low ferritin and a raised total iron binding capacity). In the developed world, IDA is usually secondary to chronic blood loss from gastrointestinal, uterine and urinary tract sources. (Worldwide hookworm infection and schistosomiasis are common causes.) In cases where the source of bleeding is obvious, further investigation is usually not necessary, and treatment can begin; however, in many instances bleeding goes unnoticed and is secondary to a more sinister cause such as gastrointestinal malignancy. As such, patients with IDA without an obvious cause must be referred for investigation of the upper and lower gastrointestinal tract in the first instance.

To treat IDA the underlying cause must be corrected and iron stores replenished. The most appropriate method of replacing iron is with oral supplementation (e.g. ferrous sulphate 200 mg TDS). Haemoglobin should rise by 1 g/dL every 7–14 days. Treatment is given until haemoglobin concentrations return to normal and for a further 3–6 months in order to replenish the depleted iron stores. If the haemoglobin fails to respond as expected, you must consider non-compliance with treatment, malabsorption and misdiagnosis. Intramuscular and intravenous preparations of iron do exist but are usually reserved for cases of refractory anaemia secondary to malabsorption and chronic disease. Blood transfusion should only be considered in severe and symptomatic anaemia (e.g. Hb <8 g/dL). The haemoglobin concentration typically increases by 1 g/dL per unit of red blood cells given.

34. ACE inhibitors

C. Renal artery stenosis

Angiotensin-converting enzyme inhibitors (ACEis) are interesting drugs which can have both renal-protective and -toxic effects. They are recommended in hypertensive patients and slow progression of renal disease by reducing systemic vascular resistance. If, however, the pathology lies with reduced renal perfusion primarily following hypovolaemia or renal artery stenosis, then ACEis will have damaging effects, as they reduce efferent blood flow further. Glomerulonephritis and lupus nephritis are both auto-immune in origin, and aside from supportive measures and renoprotection with drugs including ACEis, immunosuppression is commonly used and works with varying effect. Systemic sclerosis can affect the afferent arterioles with fibrinoid thickening and vessel narrowing, which can come on rapidly ("scleroderma renal crisis"). Immunosuppression is often unhelpful, whereas ACEis are of immense benefit and can halt progression of loss of renal function and sometimes even partially reverse it.

35. Microbiology

D. Gram-positive coccus

Staphylococcus aureus is a facultative anaerobe, i.e. it can survive without using oxygen in its metabolism but will make use of it when available. Gram-negative cocci include *Neisseria gonorrhoea* and *Neisseria meningitides*. Gram-negative rods include *Escherichia coli, Salmonella* species, *Haemophilus influenzae, Pseudomonas aeruginosa, Enterobacter* species and *Helicobacter pylori*. Gram-positive rods include *Clostridium* species and *Listeria*, whereas Gram-positive cocci of human significance are either staphylococci or streptococci. Many staphylococci are commonly found on the skin flora in humans and can cause cellulitis and intravenous line and wound infections. Initial appearance of bacteria upon Gram staining (positive or negative, cocci or rods) can, together with the clinical picture, suggest likely organisms and guide empirical antibiotic therapies before culture and sensitivities have been performed.

Staphylococcus, from Greek *staphyle* = bunch of grapes
(reference to the clumping of cocci)

36. Skin lesions

B. Basal cell carcinoma

The rolled edge, pearly appearance and telangiectasia are all classic features of basal cell carcinoma, of which there are superficial, nodular, morphoeic and basosquamous varieties. The history of sun exposure creates concerns of skin cancer. It is not described as melanocytic; therefore malignant melanoma seems highly unlikely (although amelanocytic malignant melanomas exist). Squamous cell carcinomas are ill-defined keratotic nodules that often ulcerate more so than basal cell carcinomas (BCCs). They can grow faster than the slow-growing BCCs. The risk factors are largely the same, however, and the combined investigation and management of both is simple: excise and send for histology (usually curative and diagnostic). Keratoacanthomas are rapidly growing benign tumours that often mimic squamous cell carcinomas. They can become quite large and typically develop a central ulceration and necrosis pattern. They should be excised to exclude squamous cell carcinoma, as it is difficult to tell the two apart, although many resolve spontaneously. Actinic keratoses are small, erythematous, silver-scaled patches or papules that are common in sun damage but are benign and can be treated (if sufficiently large to warrant treatment) by cryotherapy or, if diffuse, can be treated by topical 5-fluorouracil cream or imiquimod cream to save repeated cryotherapy and associated minor scarring. They have the potential to turn into squamous cell carcinomas after several years.

37. Diagnosis of abdominal pain

A. Biliary colic

Biliary colic is a localised inflammation of the gallbladder due to gallstones. The gallstone typically becomes lodged in Hartmann's pouch at the transition of the gallbladder and cystic duct. The name itself is a misnomer, as the pain is rarely "colicky" in nature, but more likely to be a severe and constant pain that may be related to the ingestion of fatty foods. Pain occurs following the consumption of fatty foods, as it is these foods which stimulate cholecystokinin (CCK) release from the I cells of the duodenum, which in turn stimulates gallbladder contraction. Gallstones typically present in patients with the 5 Fs – fat, forty, female, fair (Caucasian) and fertile (premenopausal). Management is by removal of the gallbladder (cholecystectomy), usually performed laparoscopically.

38. Ankylosing spondylitis

C. Pain present on waking in the early morning

Ankylosing spondylitis (AS) is an inflammatory disorder of the back that is more common in males. Patients present with lower back pain and stiffness of insidious onset that is worse in the morning and gets better with exercise. There is poor spinal flexion, and in severe cases patients develop a rigid lower spine with a hunch (known as the "question mark posture" or "hang dog posture"). AS may also affect the large joints asymmetrically such as knees and hips (although it affects the lumbar joints symmetrically). AS is associated with a number of extra-articular features that are remembered by the five A's: apical lung fibrosis, anterior uveitis, Achilles tendonitis/plantar fasciitis, aortic regurgitation and amyloidosis.

This diagnosis of AS is made using Schober's test: two fingers are placed 10 cm apart on the lower back of the patient (5 cm above and below the L5 vertebra in the midline), and the patient is asked to flex. An increase between the fingers of <5 cm indicates spinal stiffness. X-ray of the hip shows blurred margins of the sacroiliac joints (sacroiliitis). Characteristic radiological features of the spine in AS include erosion of the corners of the vertebral bodies (Romanus lesions), the development of bony spurs (syndesmophytes) and calcification of the spinal ligaments (bamboo spine). Treatment options in AS are physiotherapy, exercise and slow-release NSAIDs, e.g. indomethacin. Steroids, disease-modifying anti-rheumatic drugs (DMARDs) and biological agents may also be considered under the care of a rheumatologist. Most patients manage to lead a normal life, although severe cases may impair ventilation.

AS is an example of a seronegative spondyloarthropathy – diseases associated with HLA-B27 that are characterised by a lack of rheumatoid factor (hence "seronegative"). Other spondyloarthropathies are psoriatic arthritis, Reiter disease and enteropathic arthritis. The HLA-DR4 genotype is associated with rheumatoid arthritis and type 1 diabetes mellitus, but not AS.

Ankylosing spondylitis originates from the Greek *ankylos* = bent + *spondylos* = vertebra

39. Mitral stenosis

C. Double impulse apex beat

Mitral stenosis occurs as a result of a chronic autoimmune attack upon the mitral valves (triggered by group A *Streptococcus* antibodies). This leads to scar tissue formation, which ultimately tethers the leaflets and prevents them from opening fully. Mitral stenosis leads to reduced diastolic filling of the left ventricle, reduced cardiac output and hence peripheral cyanosis. It may also lead to atrial fibrillation, pulmonary hypertension and congestive heart failure. The apex beat is described as "tapping" because of the increased force in closing the mitral valve. The opening snap in diastole correlates to forced opening of the valve and may be followed by a mid-diastolic murmur. Mitral stenosis leads to left atrial enlargement, and this is related to a bifid P-wave (P mitrale) on the ECG. The P-wave is bifid due to the presence of a larger P-wave (left atrium) superimposed on a smaller one (right atrium). Hypertrophic obstructive cardiomyopathy leads to a double impulse apex beat. Treatment options typically include mitral valve replacement or valvuloplasty.

40. Management of facial weakness

C. Steroids

This man appears to have Bell palsy – an idiopathic seventh nerve palsy. The fact that the forehead is not spared means that there is lower motor neurone weakness, and the lack of any other neurological symptoms, conditions such as diabetes and vasculitis, or identifiable structural lesion along the path of the seventh nerve means that the cause is most likely to be idiopathic. It is thought to be an inflammatory process in most cases, causing compression at the facial canal or stylomastoid foramen. Steroids are commonly used in therapy, as many studies have shown greater chance of return of facial nerve function when compared to conservative management. Antiviral therapy is considered on an individual basis. A dangerous complication of Bell palsy is corneal abrasions, which can happen especially during sleep, and therefore eye protection with lubricant and an eye patch are recommended if the patient cannot close their affected eye. Therefore whilst antiretrovirals and eye protection can be used in the treatment of the disease, answer C is correct, as all patients presenting within 72 hours of symptom onset should be prescribed steroids. Penicillin-based antibiotics are used in Lyme disease, which is a rare cause of seventh nerve palsy, but there is no evidence of it here (i.e. preceding rash, arthralgia or flu-like symptoms). There is no evidence that this man's symptoms were due to an ischaemic event – the onset over a few days, lack of risk factors and lack of other neurology make this evident – and thus aspirin, dipyridamole, statin therapy and an angiotensin-converting enzyme (ACE) inhibitor would all be inappropriate.

Charles Bell, Scottish anatomist (1774-1842)

41. Pathological fracture

C. Multiple myeloma

In multiple myeloma there is malignant proliferation of plasma cells that secrete monoclonal antibodies and light immunoglobulin chains. Multiple myeloma is a multisystem disease that affects the bone marrow, skeletal system and kidneys primarily. It may also affect the heart secondary to amyloidosis. One may present with lethargy secondary to anaemia, signs of hypercalcaemia, bone pain and pathological fractures, spinal cord compression, sepsis or acute renal failure. Diagnosis requires clonal bone marrow plasma cells >10% or biopsy-proven bony or extramedullary plasmacytoma and any one or more of the following CRAB features and myeloma-defining events. The original CRAB criteria for the diagnosis of multiple myeloma (evidence of end-organ damage that can be attributed to the underlying plasma cell proliferative disorder specifically) include the following: hyper-Calcemia: serum calcium >0.25 mmol/L (>1 mg/dL) higher than the upper limit of normal or >2.75 mmol/L (>11 mg/dL); Renal insufficiency: creatinine clearance <40 mL per minute or serum creatinine >177 micro mol/L (>2 mg/dL); Anaemia: haemoglobin value of >20 g/L below the lowest limit of normal or a haemoglobin value <100 g/L; Bone lesions: one or more osteolytic lesion on skeletal radiography, CT, or positron emission tomography (PET/CT). If bone marrow has <10% clonal plasma cells, more than one bone lesion is required to distinguish from solitary plasmacytoma with minimal marrow involvement. New diagnostic criteria define the CRAB criteria as any one or more of the following biomarkers of malignancy or myeloma-defining events (MDEs): 60% or greater clonal plasma cells on bone marrow examination or serum involved/uninvolved free light chain ratio of 100 or greater, provided the absolute level of the involved light chain is at least 100 mg/L (a patient's involved free light chain, either kappa or lambda, is the one that is above the normal reference range; the uninvolved free light chain is the one that is typically in or below the normal range) or more than one focal lesion on MRI that is at least 5 mm or greater in size.

People who have evidence of serum or urine monoclonal antibodies but do not fulfil the criteria for multiple myeloma are said to have "monoclonal gammopathy of uncertain significance", which has a 2% annual risk of transforming into multiple myeloma. The treatment of multiple myeloma aims to improve symptoms and suppress disease activity. Bone pain may be controlled with analgesia, bisphosphonates, radiotherapy and orthopaedic intervention. Renal failure, caused by the deposition of light chains within the kidney, is usually managed by promoting fluid intake, although renal replacement therapy may be required. Infection, anaemia and bleeding caused by pancytopenia secondary to marrow infiltration can be managed with broad-spectrum antimicrobials, erythropoietin therapy and blood product replacement, respectively.

In patients younger than 55 years of age, allogeneic stem cell transplantation offers a hope of cure but has a treatment-related mortality rate of 30% and is associated with significant morbidity from treatment-related side effects. Chemotherapy (e.g. melphalan and prednisolone) is often used to suppress disease activity but is generally viewed as palliative. Survival is usually less than 4 years, with death occurring secondary to renal failure or infection.

Henry Bence Jones, English physician (1813-1873)

42. Management of HIV

A. All patients with HIV

HIV is a retrovirus which infects the human immune cells, particularly CD4 T lymphocytes. It uses reverse transcriptase to convert RNA to DNA, which then integrates into the host genome and replicates. HIV progresses through several stages before becoming AIDS. New guidelines from the British HIV Association (BHIVA) demonstrate that highly active antiretroviral therapy (HAART) should be started for all patients with confirmed HIV regardless of stage, as it helps patients to live longer and reduces the risk of transmission. HAART typically involves two nucleoside analogue reverse transcriptase inhibitors (NRTIs), such as zidovudine and didanosine, and one of either a protease inhibitor such as indinavir or a non-nucleoside reverse transcriptase inhibitor (NNRTI) such as efavirenz. Viral load alone, however, does not as accurately predict the onset of opportunistic infection and thus should not guide treatment. A CD4 count of <200 cells/mm^3 was previously an indication for starting HAART; however, now it is felt that starting treatment earlier before the onset of AIDS improves prognosis. One should also ensure vaccinations are fully up to date and patients are treated for any AIDS-defining illness such as invasive candidiasis, Kaposi sarcoma, toxoplasmosis and cytomegalovirus retinitis.

43. Tetralogy of Fallot

C. His pulse exhibits a radiofemoral delay

Radiofemoral delay is a symptom of coarctation of the aorta, when the coarctation (narrowing) occurs between the left subclavian artery and the aortic bifurcation. A stenosis higher up between the right brachiocephalic artery and the left subclavian artery can cause asymmetric radial pulses (still with right radiofemoral delay).

Tetralogy of Fallot has four defining malformations:

1. Ventricular septal defect (VSD).
2. Pulmonary stenosis that turns the VSD into a right–left shunt, causing cyanosis; acute attacks (due to increases in pulmonary vascular resistance) can be managed by squatting, which raises peripheral vascular resistance and therefore reduces the right–left shunt.
3. Right ventricular hypertrophy.
4. Overriding aorta, i.e. the aorta is connected to both ventricles and in this sense acts like a second VSD, above which it sits.

Etienne-Louis Arthur Fallot, French physician (1850-1911)

44. Investigation of dysphagia

D. Endoscopy

Dysphagia can be caused by a wide variety of diseases. One must consider obstructive causes such as oesophageal/stomach/head and neck malignancy, strictures following reflux/infection and post-cricoid webs. Other differentials include pharyngeal pouch, CREST syndrome and external compression from mediastinal lesions, including a large left atrium or lung malignancy. One must also consider the possibility of neurological dysfunction, including achalasia, stroke, Parkinson's disease and motor neurone disease. This man requires an endoscopy to rule out malignancy given his 4-month history coupled with signs of melaena. The other tests described can supplement the endoscopy.

45. Thalassaemia trait

E. No treatment required

Thalassaemia is an autosomal recessive disorder affecting the structure of haemoglobin (Hb). Normally Hb has two alpha and two beta chains; however, this is disrupted in thalassaemia, which in turn may lead to anaemia and reduced O_2 carrying capacity of Hb. When both genes are defective, individuals may suffer from anaemia, infections following spleen function disruption and abnormal bone structure/osteoporosis. Such patients are also at risk of iron overload with resultant damage to the heart, brain and liver following the regular blood transfusions they often require.

In this case, the patient has only inherited one thalassaemia gene and is therefore a carrier of the trait. Investigations will show a microcytic hypochromic anaemia with normal ferritin and serum iron, and there will be an increase in A2 haemoglobin on electrophoresis. It is important to differentiate thalassaemia from iron-deficiency anaemia, which may require further investigation in a man of his age. The importance of diagnosis of the thalassaemia trait is to allow genetic counselling.

46. Warfarin therapy

B. Erythromycin

Warfarin is a common anticoagulant that works by inhibiting an essential step in the synthesis of vitamin K–dependent clotting factors (II, VII, IX and X). Anticoagulation is measured using the prothrombin time (PT), which is converted into the international normalised ratio (INR) using the following formula:

$$INR = (\text{measured PT}/\text{normal PT})^{ISI}$$

where the international sensitivity index (ISI) is a constant number that represents how the particular manufactured batch of tissue factor used in the lab compares to an internationally standardised sample. It is usual for patients on warfarin to have a target INR of 2–4.5 depending on the condition being treated. Warfarin therapy is complicated, and some patients develop an inappropriately high INR, which places them at increased risk of bleeding. The most common causes for developing an inappropriately high INR are dosing errors, accidental overdose and drug interaction. Degradation of warfarin is via cytochrome p450 in the liver, which is a common pathway for many other drugs and is also susceptible to inhibition and enhancement. Drugs that are known to potentiate the action of warfarin include antibiotics (including erythromycin), sodium valproate and fluconazole. In this case it is likely that the antibiotics prescribed for the chest infection increased the action of warfarin, causing a significant rise in INR, which placed the patient at risk of a major bleed from minor trauma. The treatment of an inappropriately high INR depends on the specific circumstances. A moderately high INR with no bleeding can usually be corrected by omitting a dose of warfarin. In situations when the INR is significantly raised without bleeding, the warfarin should be omitted and an oral dose of vitamin K prescribed. A high INR associated with active bleeding warrants a dose of oral or intravenous vitamin K plus the administration of a prothrombin complex concentrate such as Beriplex, which contains the deficient factors II, VII, IX and X. When a prothrombin complex concentrate is not available, fresh frozen plasma may be used as an alternative. One must always ensure to check INR pre-operatively to ensure <1.5 and thus safe for surgery. Vitamin K can be given if required.

Warfarin, named after the Wisconsin Alumni Research Foundation, where it was discovered (Warf) + *arin* (indicating its link with coumarin, the natural compound used to make dicoumarol, another anticoagulant)

47. The painful joint

C. Bloods including FBC, UE, CRP and urate, blood cultures, XR, discussion with registrar regarding washout in theatre

The main differentials for acute swollen knee include septic arthritis, gout, pseudo gout, osteo/rheumatoid arthritis, meniscal injury, anterior cruciate ligament (ACL) rupture, extensor tendon injury and malignancy. This man is clinically well with regard to his observations. He will require a full workup to theatre washout, including bloods and knee X-ray (XR). The knee should not be aspirated on the ward and must be washed out in theatre under sterile conditions. As he is clinically well, antibiotics should be held until post-washout as microscopy, culture and Gram stain will provide antibiotic sensitivity.

48. The unresponsive patient

E. Naloxone

This man appears to be haemodynamically stable and there is no concern that that is about to change, so the fluid challenge may be unnecessary. Running some maintenance fluids for now may be indicated, as it is not known how long he may be in a coma. A blood sugar reading of 6 is normal so there is no need for the glucose. His temperature is normal, and whilst it is easy to become cold in the resuscitation room, a Bair hugger is not indicated. Flumazenil is an antidote for benzodiazepines; however, it is only used if a witnessed over-administration of benzodiazepines occurs or if respiratory depression happens secondary to benzodiazepines – reversal of benzodiazepine action can precipitate seizures or ventricular arrhythmias, and in those patients with a history of seizures, flumazenil must never be used. With this patient, it seems likely that he has taken an opioid overdose – he has pinpoint pupils and a reduced respiratory rate. Boluses of naloxone 0.8–2 mg intravenously every 2 minutes, titrating to patient response, would be indicated and could induce a rapid reversal of conscious level. Due to the half-life of naloxone being shorter than morphine, an infusion of naloxone should be considered. The patient should be referred to psychiatric liaison services and offered support with the drug and alcohol team.

49. Vomiting

C. Physiological posseting

Physiological posseting, or the effortless regurgitation of food, is a normal phenomenon in most newborn children. It is especially common in premature babies. Five percent of children will still be doing this at 12 months of age. The reassuring features in this case to rule out the other diagnoses is that he is maintaining his growth trajectory and is well in himself. Failure to thrive or being unwell in himself would be the biggest indicator that this is not normal physiological regurgitation.

50. Weight loss

A. Anorexia nervosa

Weight loss in a young girl can herald the start of a malabsorption syndrome or hormonal disturbance such as hyperthyroidism. Every case needs to be treated thoroughly, and a detailed history and investigation should point towards either organic or psychological illness. Anorexia nervosa is a common condition and is thought to have both genetic and environmental influences. A careful psychological and food history is necessary for diagnosis, especially as associated psychiatric illness such as depression and anxiety are commonplace. Treatment depends on the severity of the illness; however, the aim is to gradually restore normal weight and treat any underlying psychiatric illness. The patient should be referred to a psychiatrist specialising in eating disorders and may be offered family/cognitive behavioural therapy. Hospitalisation may be required in severe cases. An ECG should be performed to look for any heart strain, and a bone scan may be indicated if anorexia lasts for longer than 1 year to rule out osteoporosis.

Practice paper 2: Questions

1. Head trauma

Which of the following is NOT an indication for an immediate (within an hour) head CT scan after head trauma?

A Signs of basal skull fracture
B Two episodes of vomiting
C GCS 14 on initial assessment
D Seizures
E Depressed skull fracture

2. HLA-B27

Which of the following conditions is NOT associated with HLA-B27?

A Crohn's disease
B Psoriasis
C Scleritis
D Ulcerative colitis
E Uveitis

3. Heart failure

A 69-year-old man presents with a range of signs and symptoms that give the impression of heart failure.

Which of the following is NOT a feature of heart failure?

A Hepatomegaly
B Non-pitting oedema
C Pulsus alternans
D Raised jugular venous pressure
E Tricuspid regurgitation

4. Scoring systems

A 57-year-old man with a history of alcohol abuse presents with a 12-hour history of severe central epigastric pain radiating through to the back. Blood tests reveal a normal white cell count, amylase 2250 U/mL, LDH 530 IU/L, calcium 2.2 mmol/L, albumin 38 g/dL, urea 12 mmol/L and blood glucose 14 mmol/L. An arterial blood gas reading demonstrates a pO_2 of 10.2 kPa on room air.

DOI: 10.1201/9781003648222-3

What is his Glasgow score?

A 0   D 3
B 1   E 4
C 2

5. Investigation of headache

A 60-year-old man presents with total visual loss in his left eye that developed over 1 day. He says he had a headache on the left side in the 5 days that preceded the visual loss, which was constant and severe and worse on talking or eating. On further questioning he said he has been feeling lethargic for the last 2 months and has been having some shoulder aches. There is no relevant past medical history, and he has never smoked. On examination, there is no vision in the left eye, there is a relative afferent papillary defect, and the optic disc appears red and swollen on ophthalmoscopy. There is no other cranial nerve defect or neurological defect.

Which investigation would confirm the most likely diagnosis?

A Computed tomography (CT)
B Inflammatory markers (C-reactive protein [CRP], erythrocyte sedimentation rate [ESR])
C Lumbar puncture
D Temporal artery biopsy
E Visual evoked potentials

6. Management of hypercalcaemia

A 70-year-old man presents to the emergency department with a cough productive of blood-stained green sputum and shortness of breath. A chest X-ray demonstrates a suspicious lesion in the right lower zone associated with consolidation. On further questioning, he admits to recent weight loss and back pain. Blood tests show the following:

Na^+	137 mmol/L	Corrected Ca^{2+}	3.0 mmol/L
K^+	3.8 mmol/L	PO_4	0.33 mmol/L
Urea	14.5 mmol/L	Alk Phos	450 mmol/L
Creatinine	160 μmol/L		

Which of the following is NOT appropriate in the management of this patient?

A Check patient's urea and electrolyte level and serum calcium level twice daily
B Consider starting intravenous bisphosphonate
C Consider starting loop diuretics
D Rehydration with intravenous normal saline
E Request an urgent isotope bone scan

7. Shortness of breath

A 45-year-old woman with type 1 diabetes and rheumatoid arthritis has been admitted after a massive overdose of ibuprofen and has been noted to have acute renal failure with a creatinine level of around 350 µmol/L. The next day, you are called to see her, as she is becoming breathless. Her airway is clear. She looks anxious. Her respiratory rate is 28/min, and her saturations are 86% on air. You hear bibasal crepitations in her chest, which is slightly dull to percussion at both bases. She has a pulse of 110 bpm and blood pressure of 125/80 mmHg. Her urine output has been 120 ml in the last 10 hours, and you note that her jugular venous pressure is high. It appears from the notes that the night house officer was asked to see her due to her low urine output and prescribed aggressive fluid resuscitation of 3 litres over the course of 12 hours.

What is the most likely reason for her breathlessness?

A Acute respiratory distress syndrome
B Aspiration
C Pleural effusion
D Pneumonia
E Pulmonary oedema

8. Nosebleeds

A 55-year-old man is referred to haematology with repeated nosebleeds, malaise, weight loss, left upper quadrant (LUQ) abdominal pain and night sweats. Investigations show a raised white cell count, mainly neutrophils and myelocytes; anaemia; increased urate; and increased alkaline phosphatase. On blood film there are no blast cells. Genetic studies show a t(9:22) translocation encoding for the BCR-ABL gene.

What is his diagnosis?

A Acute lymphoblastic leukaemia
B Acute myeloid leukaemia
C Chronic lymphoblastic leukaemia
D Chronic myeloid leukaemia
E Non-Hodgkin lymphoma

9. Haematemesis

A 48-year-old man is admitted to the emergency department vomiting blood. He has a blood pressure of 80/45 mmHg with a heart rate of 135 bpm. He is cool and clammy to the touch.

Which of the following should NOT be in your immediate management of this patient?

A Alert the endoscopy suite
B Contact senior support
C Crossmatch 6–8 U blood urgently
D Insert two large-bore cannulae
E Transfer to the ward

10. Failure to thrive

A 5-month-old girl presents with failure to thrive, pallor and mild jaundice. The child has frontal bossing of the skull, prominent maxillae and hepatosplenomegaly.

Which of the following is the most likely diagnosis?

A Congenital biliary atresia
B Congenital hypothyroid
C Hydrops fetalis
D Lead poisoning
E Thalassaemia major

11. Osteoarthritis of the hand

Which of the following findings on hand examination are suggestive of osteoarthritis?

A Dactylitis
B Osteophytes at the distal and/or proximal interphalangeal joints
C Prominent nail fold capillary loops
D Prominent ulnar styloid
E Trigger finger

12. Study design

Several trials have been published regarding the role of therapeutic statin use in bowel cancer. The published results are disparate, and you wish to find the best answer from the available literature.

Which of the following study designs would you use?

A Case series
B Delphi method
C Meta-analysis
D Non-systematic review
E Randomised, controlled trial

13. Hand infection

A 35-year-old male with a history of type 1 diabetes attends the accident and emergency department with a 12-hour history of a painful, swollen right index finger. He is not aware of any direct trauma but does bite his nails. On examination his index finger is grossly swollen and slightly flexed with pain on passive extension. His observations demonstrate a slight tachycardia of 105 bpm.

What is the most likely diagnosis?

A Flexor tenosynovitis
B Paronychia
C Felon

D Cellulitis
E Necrotising fasciitis

14. Mouth ulcers

A 29-year-old woman is concerned about recurrent ulcers she gets in her mouth. Occurring every few months, they are small, grey, shallow ulcers that disappear spontaneously. She has no other gastrointestinal symptoms or weight loss.

What is the most likely cause?

A Behçet disease
B Crohn's disease
C Herpes simplex

D Idiopathic aphthous ulcers
E Oral carcinoma

15. Antibiotics

From the following list of antibiotics and their predominant cover, which is incorrect?

A Co-amoxiclav – broad-spectrum Gram-positive and Gram-negative cover
B Flucloxacillin – Gram-positive cover
C Gentamicin – Gram-negative cover
D Metronidazole – anaerobic cover
E Vancomycin – Gram-negative cover

16. Pleural effusion

A 62-year-old Asian woman presents to the emergency department with increasing shortness of breath for the past 2 weeks. She has a past medical history of breast cancer, ischaemic heart disease, previous myocardial infarction with a stent in her left anterior descending artery, and osteoarthritis. On examination, there are reduced breath sounds on her lung bases and dullness to percussion. Both legs are swollen. A chest X-ray demonstrates a right-sided pleural effusion. A simple aspiration of the pleural cavity showed a pleural fluid protein: serum protein ratio <0.5.

What is the most likely underlying diagnosis?

A Congestive cardiac failure
B Metastatic lung cancer
C Rheumatoid disease
D Systemic lupus erythematosus
E Tuberculosis

17. Topical steroids

A 25-year-old man presents with a severe outbreak of a dry, erythematous, itchy rash that is now widespread, despite having used a steroid cream prescribed by his GP. It appears to be eczema, and along with regular emollients for the dryness and antihistamines for the itch, you would like to prescribe some very potent topical steroids for a brief period to attempt get on top of the outbreak.

Which of the following is classed as a very potent topical steroid?

A Betnovate
B Dermovate
C Eumovate
D Hydrocortisone
E Prednisolone

18. Skin lesion

A 7-year-old boy presents with multiple erythematous patches over both sides of his face, head, neck, upper chest and left arm and shoulder, which appear to be covered in a honey-coloured crust. His mother says that the lesions have spread over about a week, starting at the left neck and radiating outwards. The child appears to be upset, and the lesions are itchy. There is past medical history and no history of recent infections.

Which of the following diagnoses is most likely?

A Eczema
B Erysipelas
C Impetigo
D Psoriasis
E Staphylococcal scalded skin syndrome

19. Management of Parkinson's disease

A 75-year-old man has been recently diagnosed with Parkinson's disease and started on levodopa (L-DOPA), which has helped his tremor and bradykinesia significantly. However, in the past week he had a fall shortly after getting out of his chair, during which he briefly blacked out and afterwards was sweating and felt cold.

Which of the following side effects most likely explains the fall?

A Dyskinesia
B Hallucinations
C Nausea
D None; he actually has multiple system atrophy and not Parkinson's disease
E Postural hypotension

20. Arrhythmias

You are reviewing the medication of a 62-year-old man suffering from depression and cardiac arrhythmias. He was recently discharged from hospital for chest pain. During his admission, he was noted to have "torsades de pointes".

What is torsades de pointes?

A A clinical sign associated with acute pericarditis
B A congenital facial sign associated with congenital heart defects
C A form of ventricular tachycardia that can self-correct but can also lead to sudden death
D A variation in the QRS that changes in magnitude with inspiration and expiration
E Alternate T-wave inversion

21. Back pain

A 69-year-old man recently diagnosed with metastatic prostate cancer presents with weakness in his legs and urinary retention. He has had back pain for years but in the last 24 hours this has become very severe in his lower back. On examination he has a sensory deficit, loss of anal tone and poor sensation in the skin around the anus. When catheterised he has a residual volume of 1.5 L.

Which of the following is the most informative initial investigation?

A Computed tomography (CT) of the abdomen/pelvis
B Lumbar X-rays
C Magnetic resonance imaging (MRI) of the whole spine
D Serum calcium
E Ultrasound scan (USS) of the renal tract

22. Bruising in children

A 6-year-old boy has a 1-month history of aching bones and muscle pains. On examination he appears pale and has multiple bruises along his legs. He has extensive lymphadenopathy. Blast cells are seen on the blood film.

What is the most likely diagnosis?

A Acute lymphoblastic leukaemia
B Child abuse
C Henoch–Schönlein purpura
D Juvenile idiopathic arthritis
E Sickle cell disease

23. Management of skin lesions

A 76-year-old man presents with a vesicular eruption on the left side of his forehead only. It is severely painful, and the vesicles have started to crust over. On examination, the affected area is well-demarcated. You also note a red eye with apparent conjunctivitis.

Given the most likely diagnosis, which of the following treatments is the most appropriate?

A Intravenous steroids
B Oral or IV aciclovir pending ophthalmology review
C Topical aciclovir
D Topical antibiotic
E Topical steroids

24. Coarctation of the aorta

You find a loud systolic murmur in a 14-year-old girl during a preoperative assessment for an appendicectomy.

Which of the following signs or investigations do NOT help confirm a diagnosis of coarctation of the aorta?

A Ankle–brachial pressure index
B Electrocardiogram
C Magnetic resonance angiography
D Radial pulse asymmetry
E Radiofemoral delay

25. Management of asthma

A 28-year-old woman with a past medical history of asthma has been using her inhaled salbutamol more frequently of late. She is currently on an inhaled short-acting beta-2 agonist and an inhaled steroid 800 µg/day. She has been compliant.

What should you do?

A Add an inhaled long-acting beta-2 agonist
B Prescribe a short-acting muscarinic antagonist
C Add an oral steroid
D Increase the dose of inhaled steroid
E Prescribe an inhaled short-acting beta-2 agonist as regular therapy

26. Collapse

A 62-year-old woman presents to the emergency department with collapse. She felt dizzy when she tried to stand up from a sitting position. She did not lose consciousness. She denied any visual disturbances, headache or head injury. She also complained of fatigue over the past month. She takes only omeprazole and paracetamol. An electrocardiogram (ECG) showed normal sinus rhythm. Her blood pressure was 102/50 mmHg. A blood test revealed the following: Na^+ 126 mmol/L, K^+ 6.5 mmol/L, urea 10.0 mmol/L and creatinine 139 μmol/L.

What is the most likely diagnosis?

A Acromegaly
B Adrenal insufficiency
C Cushing's disease
D Hypocalcaemia
E Hypothyroidism

27. Diagnosis of abdominal pain

A 56-year-old man with a long history of alcohol abuse presents to the emergency department with abdominal pain. On examination he has a distended abdomen with shifting dullness and has a temperature of 38.2°C.

What is the most likely diagnosis?

A Bowel obstruction
B Liver cirrhosis
C Mallory–Weiss syndrome
D Perforated peptic ulcer
E Spontaneous bacterial peritonitis (SBP)

28. Investigation of stroke

A 52-year-old man with hyperthyroidism, vitiligo and a 30-pack/year smoking history presents to hospital with an acute clumsiness of his right hand. Neurological examination reveals normal cranial nerves, and the only abnormal feature on the limb examination is some past pointing and dysdiadochokinesis in the right hand. Diffusion-weighted magnetic resonance imaging (MRI) reveals a small right-sided cerebellar infarct.

Which of the following investigations is unlikely to be helpful?

A Carotid Doppler
B Electrocardiogram (ECG)
C Erythrocyte sedimentation rate (ESR)
D Full blood count
E Magnetic resonance angiography

29. Diagnosis of cough

A 32-year-old woman originally from Jamaica presents to the GP with a 3-month history of nonproductive cough and breathlessness on exertion. She also complains of fatigue, weight loss and joint pain. She smokes 15 cigarettes a day. She has not travelled to any foreign countries recently. On examination, fine interstitial crackles are heard on the anterior chest wall. There are multiple tender red lumps on both shins.

What is the most likely diagnosis?

A Idiopathic pulmonary fibrosis
B Lung cancer
C Sarcoidosis
D Systemic lupus erythematosus
E Wegener granulomatosis

30. Diagnosis of multiple sclerosis

Which of the following findings on lumbar puncture is most commonly used to suggest a diagnosis of multiple sclerosis, given a correlative clinical picture?

A Autoantibodies to myelin basic protein
B Oligoclonal bands on electrophoresis
C Presence of red blood cells
D Raised lymphocytes
E Raised protein

31. Investigation of abdominal pain

A 59-year-old woman with known polycythaemia vera presents to the emergency department with right upper quadrant pain, tender hepatomegaly and gross ascites, which has come on suddenly. There is no jaundice.

What is the next most appropriate investigation?

A Cytomegalovirus (CMV) screen
B Gamma-glutamyl transferase (GGT) levels
C Hepatitis serology
D Hepatic vein Doppler ultrasound scan (USS)
E Human immunodeficiency virus (HIV) testing

32. Diagnosis of cough

A 60-year-old Chinese man presents to the GP with a 4-month history of weight loss. He has lost around 1 stone in weight. He also has a cough productive of green sputum without blood. He has a reduced appetite, insomnia and night sweats. His past medical history includes hypertension and ischaemic heart disease. He is a retired managing director who has just emigrated from Hong Kong to England. He denies a smoking history. His observations include temperature 36.4°C, pulse 67 bpm, blood pressure 152/92 mmHg and respiratory rate 15/min. On examination, there is dullness to percussion over the left upper lung zone.

What is the most likely diagnosis?

A Lung cancer
B Lung abscess
C Pulmonary infarction
D Tuberculosis
E Wegener granulomatosis

33. Diagnosis of tuberculosis

A 27-year-old man presents with a 3-month history of cough with some blood streaking, loss of weight and night sweats. You suspect tuberculosis.

Which of the following chest X-ray findings is NOT consistent with tuberculosis?

A Cavitating lesion
B Consolidation of a lobe
C Diffuse 1- to 2-mm spots of increased opacity
D Perihilar ground-glass changes
E Pleural effusion

34. Thrombocytopenia

A 74-year-old man is admitted to hospital with an acute-on-chronically ischaemic leg and started on intravenous heparin. Blood tests taken 5 days later show platelet levels have dropped from 250 to 54×10^9.

What is the most likely cause for thrombocytopenia in this patient?

A Chronic lymphocytic leukaemia
B Disseminated intravascular coagulation
C Evans syndrome
D Heparin-induced thrombocytopenia (HIT)
E Thrombotic thrombocytopenic purpura

35. Meningitis

A 40-year-old man presents to the emergency department after 8 hours of a severe frontal headache, photophobia and two episodes of vomiting. On examination his Glasgow Coma Score (GCS) is 13 (eyes open to voice, verbal response with confused sentences and moving freely); he has a temperature of 38.5°C; a BP of 95/65 mmHg; and a pulse rate of 105 bpm. He is photophobic and has neck stiffness. There is no rash and no focal neurological deficit as far as you can ascertain. His wife is present and is able to elaborate on the history. Since having lost his job 7 months back, he has been drinking 8–10 cans of lager per night. He has recently been coughing a lot and feels unwell. He still lives at home and has not appeared to lose weight recently.

What are you most concerned that this might be?

A *Listeria* meningitis

B Meningococcal meningitis

C Pneumococcal meningitis

D Tubercular meningitis

E Viral meningitis

36. Electrocardiogram

A 63-year-old male smoker on diuretics for essential hypertension presents to the emergency department with chest pain. His ECG is presented to you. Amongst other signs, you notice T-wave inversion.

Which of the following does not cause T-wave inversion?

A Hyperkalaemia

B Left bundle branch block

C Left ventricular hypertrophy

D Myocardial infarction

E Myocardial ischaemia

37. Diarrhoea

A 72-year-old man is bed-bound following a severe stroke several years previously and lives in a nursing home with full-time care. The staff noticed that over the last 8 days he didn't pass any stool motions until this morning, when there was profuse, offensive liquid stool. They are concerned this may be infective diarrhoea. On examination there is hard stool in the rectum.

What is the most likely diagnosis?

A *Campylobacter* infection

B Carcinoma of the rectum

C Inflammatory bowel disease

D Norovirus

E Overflow diarrhoea

38. Management of epilepsy

A 24-year-old man presents with two episodes of involuntary clonic beating of the right arm followed by loss of consciousness with urinary and faecal incontinence. He then had a headache and confusion for some hours (no-one witnessed any episode). A diagnosis of motor partial seizures with secondary generalisation is made. He is started on valproate.

Which of the following would you NOT tell him (as it is untrue)?

A Computed tomography (CT)/magnetic resonance imaging (MRI) is indicated to look for a cause
B No driving for 1 year after the last seizure
C On valproate, blood tests will need to be monitored for liver enzymes and full blood count
D Valproate may cause gum hypertrophy
E Valproate may cause hair loss

39. Diagnosis of HIV-related illness

A 42-year-old woman with known HIV presents with a 3-week history of dry cough and increasing breathlessness. She is now unable to walk 100 yards without becoming short of breath. You suspect *Pneumocystis* pneumonia.

Which of the following tests is the best way to confirm the diagnosis?

A Bronchoalveolar lavage
B Chest X-ray
C Computed tomography (CT) of the chest
D Cytology of sputum induced by nebulised hypertonic saline
E Hypoxaemia on arterial blood gas

40. Tiredness

A 65-year-old woman presents to her GP complaining of tiredness, shortness of breath and loss of sensation in her feet. On examination she is visibly pale and has mild jaundice and glossitis. She has loss of joint position sense and vibration distally, with extensor plantar reflexes, absent ankle jerks and brisk knee jerks bilaterally.

What is the most likely cause for her symptoms?

A Chronic sickle cell disease
B G6PD deficiency
C Heart failure
D Renal failure
E Vitamin B$_{12}$ deficiency

41. Management of acne

A 17-year-old girl shuffles awkwardly into the dermatology clinic with her mother, who explains that her daughter has suffered from severe acne for the last few years and nothing that the GP has tried has shifted it. She has tried benzoyl peroxide, azelaic acid and both topical and oral antibiotics. On examination, as well as several large pustules on her face and comedones, some scarring is beginning to develop. You would like to start oral isotretinoin (Roaccutane).

When counselling about side effects, which of the following would you NOT advise the patient?

A It commonly leads to hearing loss
B Blood tests should be taken to monitor for raised liver function tests
C People may feel depressed on isotretinoin
D Parts of the skin and lips often get very dry
E Pregnancy should be avoided, as teratogenicity is a risk

42. Epigastric pain

A 68-year-old man presents with a 3-month history of epigastric pain and weight loss. He has a history of acid reflux, which his GP has been managing. He is a long-term smoker and drinks 20 units alcohol weekly.

What is the next most appropriate step?

A Computed tomography (CT) scan of the abdomen
B Dietician review
C Increase his proton pump inhibitor (PPI) and ask him to return in 1 month if symptoms don't settle
D Treat empirically for *Helicobacter pylori* infection and review in 1 month
E Upper gastrointestinal (GI) endoscopy

43. Skin loss – new question and answer

A 56-year-old woman with type 2 diabetes, COPD, HIV and lung cancer attends her GP for antibiotics for a chest infection. Shortly after commencing clarithromycin, she starts to feel feverish and lethargic. The following morning, she subsequently notices her skin blistering over her torso. She attends accident and emergency, and on assessment the blistering is now involving >30% of her body and her oral mucosa. Her observations demonstrate hypotension and tachycardia, and her bloods indicate acute renal failure.

What is the most likely diagnosis?

A Anaphylaxis
B Stevens–Johnson syndrome
C Toxic epidermal necrolysis
D Meningitis
E Kaposi sarcoma

44. Management of DKA

A 19-year-old boy is admitted with a 3-week history of polyuria, polydipsia and lethargy. He had initially put this down to increased training sessions with his university football club. His flatmates called an ambulance this morning when they realised he had missed morning lectures and they found him drowsy in bed. Diabetic ketoacidosis (DKA) was quickly diagnosed in accident and emergency.

Which of the following is the most appropriate prescription for the insulin required as part of the treatment plan?

A Intravenous insulin at a dose of 0.1 units/kg/hour until blood glucose <14 mmol/L and then switch to 0.05 units/kg/hour

B Subcutaneous insulin at a dose of 15 units stat, and reassess need for more by checking blood glucose at 2 hours post-initial dose

C Intravenous insulin at a dose of 0.1 units/kg/hour until blood glucose <10 mmol/L and then switch to 0.05 units/kg/hour

D Subcutaneous insulin at a dose of 20 units stat, and reassess need for more by checking blood glucose at 2 hours post-initial dose

E Intravenous insulin at a dose of 10 units/kg/hour until blood glucose <14 mmol/L and then switch to 5 units/kg/hour

45. Renal transplantation

Which of the following is NOT a contraindication to renal transplantation?

A Active tuberculosis

B High-pressure urinary tract, e.g. posterior urethral valves

C Malignancy

D Severe arterial disease with stenosed iliac vessels

E Severe ischaemic heart disease with unstable angina and congestive cardiac failure

46. Thrombolysis in ischaemic stroke

Which of the following patients is eligible for thrombolysis with intravenous recombinant tissue plasminogen activator?

A 2 hours post-onset, BP 150/80 mmHg, GCS 11, MRI shows infarct

B 2 hours post-onset, BP 160/90 mmHg, GCS 15, MRI shows haemorrhage

C 2 hours post-onset, BP 160/95 mmHg, GCS 15, MRI shows infarct

D 2 hours post-onset, BP 195/115 mmHg, GCS 15, MRI shows infarct

E 7 hours post-onset, BP 135/80 mmHg, GCS 15, MRI shows infarct

47. Diagnosis of chest pain

A 43-year-old woman presents with an acute sharp, central chest pain radiating to the left arm that is worse on inspiration and at night. She reports that it is preventing her from coughing, which, in turn, is prolonging a recent chest infection. On examination, her chest exhibits vesicular breath sounds with bibasal crackles. Her electrocardiogram (ECG) shows widespread concave ST elevation in sinus rhythm.

Which of the following is the most likely diagnosis?

A Acute pericarditis
B Cardiac tamponade
C Pulmonary embolism
D ST-elevated myocardial infarction
E Unstable angina

48. Management of oliguria

An 87-year-old man with a background of Alzheimer's disease, a previous stroke and atrial fibrillation (for which he is on warfarin) is admitted with increasing amounts of painless haematuria. He is catheterised and the warfarin stopped. The haematuria reduces and then seems to stop. Problems with his residential home are delaying discharge. You note 2 days later that his creatinine level has risen to 250 μmol/L. When you go to see him, he seems stable, as do his observations. He does seem slightly dry with reduced skin turgor and delayed capillary refill. The urine output has not been carefully documented in the last few days, and by your calculations, 100 mL have been passed in the last 24 hours. On examination he appears to have a mass in his central lower abdomen.

What should be your next step?

A Fluid challenge of 500 mL normal saline over 10 minutes
B Flush the catheter with 50 mL warm saline and then aspirate
C Insert a suprapubic catheter
D Remove the catheter
E Request a CT kidneys–ureter–bladder (KUB)

49. The unresponsive patient

A 70-year-old woman presents with hip pain following a fall. The fall appears to have been related to alcohol ingestion, and whilst the history is vague, she denies loss of consciousness and does not seem grossly confused, nor is there evidence of infection. She is a smoker and has a history of ischaemic heart disease and depression. A hip fracture is ruled out, and she is admitted for rehabilitation purposes. On day 3, however, the nurses report that she is increasingly sleepy and muddled. On examination, observations are stable, she is apyrexial, her Glasgow Coma Score (GCS) is 12, and on neurological examination, she appears to have some mild left arm and leg weakness with normal or brisk reflexes. There is no hemianopia or other neurological deficit.

Which of the following is most likely to explain the changes?

A Bacterial meningitis
B Intracerebral haemorrhage
C Lacunar infarct
D Subarachnoid haemorrhage
E Subdural haematoma

50. Thyrotoxicosis

A 40-year-old woman presents to the GP with a history of weight loss and irritability. She has lost 1 stone in the past 2 weeks. She claims that she has a normal appetite. She also complains of blurring of the vision for the past month. On examination, she has a "staring look" with lid lag and lid retraction.

What is the most likely diagnosis?

A Graves' disease
B Hashimoto's thyroiditis
C Multinodular goitre
D Myasthenia gravis
E Toxic thyroid adenoma

Practice paper 2: Answers

1. Head trauma

C. GCS 14 on initial assessment

National Institute for Health and Care Excellence (NICE) CT head guidelines suggest imaging within the hour for GCS <13 on admission, <15 2 hours later, open or depressed skull fractures, basal skull fractures, seizures, focal neurology and >1 episode vomiting. If the patient is anticoagulated, >65 years in age, dangerous mechanism of injury with amnesia or loss of consciousness, then consider imaging within 8 hours.

2. HLA-B27

C. Scleritis

Inflammatory bowel disease is associated with HLA-B27, as is psoriasis. Uveitis is inflammation of the iris and associated structures and causes acute pain with blurred vision and photophobia with reddening of the iris. This is associated with both ankylosing spondylitis and HLA-B27. Scleritis is inflammation of the sclera, causing pain and a gritty sensation in the eye with redness of the sclera. This is associated with connective tissue disorders and rheumatoid arthritis. If left untreated, this can cause perforation of the eye. It is not associated with HLA-B27. Genetic testing for HLA-B27 can be useful in difficult diagnostic cases for seronegative spondyloarthropathies and in counselling patients regarding chances of their offspring developing the same disease.

3. Heart failure

B. Non-pitting oedema

Cardiac output is a product of heart rate multiplied by stroke volume. Heart failure is a disease of chronic, insidious onset that can first present with fatigue, shortness of breath, orthopnoea and paroxysmal nocturnal dyspnoea. Multiple compensatory mechanisms occur in the early stages of heart failure to maintain cardiac output; however, the disease eventually progresses. One mechanism is demonstrated by Starling's curve and how stretching of myocardium increases stroke volume initially until this

DOI: 10.1201/9781003648222-4

mechanism becomes overwhelmed. Another compensatory mechanism is an increased heart rate, which eventually leads to higher oxygen demand and failure. Finally, due to reduced cardiac output and reduced renal perfusion, the renin–angiotensin system activates, leading to increased fluid retention which ultimately increases the pre-load and strain on the heart.

Due to the nature of the disease and taking into account Starling's law, one can now appreciate how the subsequent raised end-diastolic volume causes a pre-stretched ventricle, leading to a more forceful contraction (Starling's law). This alternating strong-weak pattern can be seen in the ECG as pulsus alternans (varying amplitudes of the R-wave). A column of blood builds up proximal to the left ventricle in the lungs, causing pulmonary oedema. This creates afterload upon the right ventricle, which can lead to tricuspid regurgitation. The bottleneck of blood can extend further, through the right side of the heart, and hence jugular venous pressure (JVP) is raised (the heart is unable to pull all the blood from the jugular vein through the lungs and the left ventricle). Furthermore, close to the right side of the heart, the inferior vena cava remains full of blood, leading to oedema in the liver (hepatomegaly). Ankle veins become distended due to venous congestion, as the weakened heart is unable to effectively return blood against gravity from the lower limbs. The increased hydrostatic pressure results in fluid extravasation into tissues. The push of a finger is enough to displace this tissue fluid; hence this ankle oedema is pitting. Causes of non-pitting oedema include lymphoedema and pretibial myxoedema.

Oedema, from Greek *oedema* = swelling

4. Scoring systems

C. 2

The massively raised amylase with this clinical picture supports a diagnosis of acute pancreatitis. Acute pancreatitis can be a life-threatening condition for it is an unpredictable disease that can cause quick deterioration. To aid management, the modified Glasgow criteria were devised to help prognosis and triage patients to an appropriate level of care. The eight parts of the Glasgow criteria are as follows (1 point for each):

Age	>55 years
White cell count	$>15 \times 10^3/\mu L$
Urea	>16 mmol/L
Glucose	>10 mmol/L
Arterial pO_2	<8 kPa
Albumin	<32 mmol/L
Calcium	<2.0 mmol/L
Lactate dehydrogenase	>600 mmol/L

This man scores 2 for age and his raised blood sugar, which is a moderate risk for pancreatitis. A score of 3 and above should indicate to the physician the need to discuss the case with intensive care, as these patients are more likely to need invasive monitoring of their fluid balance. Patients should ideally be rescored 48 hours after admission.

5. Investigation of headache

D. Temporal artery biopsy

The most likely diagnosis is temporal arteritis, also known as giant cell arteritis (GCA). The preceding constant, severe headache with jaw claudication is highly characteristic. In addition, the patient may have polymyalgia rheumatica (PMR), which co-exists in approximately 20% of GCA cases. The question asks for the investigation that confirms the diagnosis, which is a temporal artery biopsy. This is the gold standard, although interpretation should be cautious due to the presence of possible skip lesions, where inflamed segments of the artery alternate with normal sections. While inflammatory markers (ESR and CRP) are typically raised and supportive of the diagnosis, they are non-specific. Visual evoked potentials may demonstrate optic nerve dysfunction but do not identify the underlying cause. Lumbar puncture is unlikely to contribute meaningfully in this context, and CT imaging is not sensitive for detecting vascular inflammation or soft tissue pathology.

6. Management of hypercalcaemia

E. Request an urgent isotope bone scan

The most common causes of hypercalcaemia are primary hyperparathyroidism and malignant hypercalcaemia. Patients with hypercalcaemia may have a varied clinical presentation but may include polyuria, polydipsia, renal colic, nausea, anorexia, lethargy, dyspepsia, peptic ulceration, constipation, depression, drowsiness and impaired cognition. Remember the phrase "bone, stones, abdominal moans and psychiatric groans". One must treat the urgent clinical problem of hypercalcaemia first before investigating in the coming days the potential reasons for the rise in calcium, which with this history will most likely discover a lung malignancy. Urgent fluid replacement with 0.9% saline is essential (3–6 L over 24 hours), and the patient's urea and electrolyte and calcium levels should be checked twice daily. Loop diuretics could aid renal clearance of calcium. Intravenous bisphosphonate (e.g. pamidronate) could cause a fall in calcium by causing bone reabsorption. Its effect is maximal at 2–3 days and lasts a few weeks.

7. Shortness of breath

E. Pulmonary oedema

Acute respiratory distress syndrome occurs when inflammatory cytokines and/or lung injury causes capillary permeability to increase and non-fluid overload–related pulmonary oedema. In this case there was no known preceding lung injury and no systemic acute precipitant such as sepsis, shock, haemorrhage or transfusion. The finding of bibasal crackles, however, is consistent with oedema, and whilst the diagnosis is not the most parsimonious, it cannot be entirely ruled out. There has been no vomiting reported to suggest aspiration. A pleural effusion would give stony, dull percussion and reduced air entry. This patient is clearly fluid overloaded and so there may be small effusions, but these are unlikely to be the chief cause of breathlessness. The patient is afebrile, and the symmetrical pattern to the crackles goes against (but needn't rule out) a pneumonia. The patient is in acute renal failure, likely secondary to a combination of the long-term use of non-steroidal anti-inflammatory drugs (NSAIDs; she has rheumatoid arthritis) and the recent NSAID overdose, with a background of diabetes. She is fluid overloaded (note the raised jugular venous pressure [JVP]), and the busy overnight house officer probably presumed the low urine output and raised creatinine level was due to dehydration (it appears they didn't read the notes fully) and thus has contributed to the situation. The bibasal crepitations are indicative of pulmonary oedema.

The patient should be placed in a sitting position and wear an oxygen mask, given an opiate such as morphine or diamorphine (to relieve anxiety and also to act as a vasodilator and pool fluid away from the lungs) and given some intravenous furosemide – 40 mg stat is a normal dose to try. Informing the registrar would be essential. Nitrates can also be used – glyceryl trinitrite (GTN) spray can be given before starting a nitrate infusion (if the systolic blood pressure is above 90 mmHg). Nitrates again act as a vasodilator and venodilator and pool blood away from the lungs. Pulmonary oedema is a common complication of acute renal failure. Once therapy is initiated, a portable chest X-ray should be ordered to confirm or deny the diagnosis. Further treatment of non-responders includes continuous positive airway pressure (CPAP), and refractory pulmonary oedema is one of the indications for haemofiltration or dialysis in acute renal failure.

8. Nosebleeds

D. Chronic myeloid leukaemia

The t(9:22) translocation (i.e. a translocation between chromosomes 9 and 22) encoding for the *BCR-ABL* gene is also known as the Philadelphia chromosome and is the genetic mutation in over 90% of the cases of chronic myeloid leukaemia. The mutation is a balanced translocation, which leads to increased tyrosine kinase activity disturbing stem cell kinetics.

Chronic myeloid leukaemia (CML) is a myeloproliferative disorder. Its peak incidence is 50–70 years, and it is rare in children. There is excessive proliferation of myeloid cells in the bone marrow. Patients typically have massive splenomegaly leading to reduced appetite and weight loss, anaemia, bruising, infection, fever and night sweats. A blood film shows myeloblasts (granulocyte precursors) and granulocytosis. Patients with CML but without the Philadelphia chromosome have a worse prognosis compared to those with the translocation. There are three stages of disease in CML: (1) the chronic phase (which is responsive to treatment), (2) the accelerated phase (where the disease is difficult to control) and (3) the blast crisis phase (where the disease progresses into an acute leukaemia, usually acute myeloblastic leukaemia [AML]). The median survival rate is 5 years. Death usually occurs within months of blast transformation (from bleeding and infection). Chemotherapy is often used, and allogeneic stem cell transplantation can provide a cure. Having isolated the gene, there is now an effective drug that can block the *BCRABL* gene – imatinib mesylate – which can reverse the effects of the protein and produce remission in 95% of patients with this mutation.

9. Haematemesis

E. Transfer to the ward

Shock is inadequate tissue perfusion and may be cardiogenic, hypovolaemic or distributive, including sepsis and anaphylaxis. This case presents a young man who is in hypovolaemic shock following a large upper gastrointestinal (GI) bleed. Haemorrhagic shock has four stages, and be aware that only in stage 3, when over 2 litres of blood (>30% blood volume) has been lost, does the blood pressure start to fall. Immediate management in these cases is vital to improving mortality, which is currently about 10% for major bleeds. The aetiology includes gastritis/duodenitis, gastric/duodenal ulcers, oesophageal varices, Mallory–Weiss tears and oesophageal/gastric malignancy. Initial management relies on effective resuscitation of the patient. Always start with ABC, securing the airway, giving supplementary oxygen, and using two large-bore cannulae to ensure rapid fluid infusion is possible. One must consider the trauma triad of hypothermia, coagulopathy and acidosis which emphasises the importance of warm fluid/blood products to enhance resuscitation. Blood products are the best resuscitative agents – always try to replace like with like. However, while you await a crossmatch use a crystalloid infusion, or O-negative blood can be given. A catheter should be inserted early during the resuscitation, as urine output is a very sensitive marker of renal perfusion. This patient needs to be in a monitored bed while he remains shocked, and so transfer to a ward would not normally be appropriate. Following resuscitation, your next actions will depend on aetiology, but if variceal bleeding is suspected, an urgent endoscopy and sclerotherapy or banding will be necessary. Alerting the necessary teams at the time of presentation can save vital minutes and ensure that you have the support you need around you.

10. Failure to thrive

E. Thalassaemia major

Beta-thalassaemia major is an autosomal recessive disorder in which there is a complete lack of production of the haemoglobin chain beta-globin. It occurs mainly in Mediterranean and Middle Eastern families and is due to a point mutation on chromosome 11. Because patients with beta-thalassaemia major have mutations on both alleles and cannot synthesise any beta-globin, they cannot produce functioning adult haemoglobin (HbA – $\alpha_2\beta_2$). This condition typically presents within the first year of life, when the production of fetal haemoglobin (HbF – $\alpha_2\gamma_2$) begins to fall. Affected children become generally unwell and fail to thrive secondary to a severe microcytic anaemia. Ferritin levels are normal since there is no iron deficiency. A compensatory increase in the synthesis of HbF and haemoglobin A2 (HbA2 – $\alpha_2\delta_2$) occurs, which can be detected on serum electrophoresis.

Clinical features include failure to thrive, lethargy, pallor and jaundice. On examination there is often hepatosplenomegaly (secondary to extramedullary haematopoiesis) with bossing of the skull, maxillary prominence and long bone deformity (due to excessive intramedullary haematopoiesis). The treatment of beta-thalassaemia major is with regular blood transfusions, aiming to maintain the haemoglobin concentration above 10 g/dL, or with allogenic bone marrow transplant. Regular iron chelation therapy (with desferrioxamine) is required to prevent iron overload and deposition in vital organs such as the heart, liver and endocrine glands. If untreated, death is inevitable in the first years of life.

Beta-thalassaemia minor describes people heterozygous for the beta-chain chromosomal mutation. Affected persons have only mild anaemia and are usually asymptomatic. Alpha-thalassaemia is common in Southeast Asia. There are four alpha genes, and therefore four variants of alpha-thalassaemia. Affected patients can be asymptomatic (one gene corruption), have mild hypochromic anaemia (two corruptions), have HbH disease (three corruptions) or can die in utero (all four genes are corrupted). HbH is a beta-chain tetramer that is functionally useless. Treatment options are as for beta-thalassaemia.

Thalassaemia, from Greek *thalassa* = sea + *haima* = blood. It is so-called, as the disease is especially prevalent in countries by the sea (i.e. the Mediterranean)

11. Osteoarthritis of the hand

B. Osteophytes at the distal and/or proximal interphalangeal joints

Dactylitis simply means inflammation of the digit(s). Dactylitis can be seen in psoriatic arthropathy – the red, swollen, tender fingers are sometimes referred to as "sausage fingers". Osteophytes at the distal interphalangeal joints are called Heberden nodes and are characteristic of osteoarthritis. Bouchard nodes are osteophytes at the proximal interphalangeal joints and usually appear later than Heberden nodes. Prominent nail fold capillary loops are one of the many skin manifestations of dermatomyositis, an inflammatory disease of the muscle that also affects the skin and is commonly paraneoplastic (i.e. related to an underlying tumour). The prominent ulnar styloid is a change seen in rheumatoid arthritis, which is caused by radial deviation at the wrist joint. Trigger finger is often seen in psoriatic arthritis and rheumatoid arthritis, and its aetiology is not entirely clear but involves disparity between the flexor tendon and its sheath, which prevents extension of the finger. The finger can suddenly snap back into extension, hence the label "trigger finger". Corticosteroid injection should be tried and is effective in many cases, failing which surgery can release the tendon from its sheath.

William Heberden, English physician (1710–1801)

Charles-Joseph Bouchard, French pathologist (1837–1915)

12. Study design

C. Meta-analysis

A meta-analysis combines the results of several studies that have looked at a similar hypothesis. By combining the results of multiple data sets, the statistical power of the outcome is increased and the validity of the conclusion improved. Case series is a type of observational study that tracks subjects with a known exposure. The Delphi method involves discussion of a topic amongst a focus group of experts in order to arrive at the most agreed-upon solution. As such, it is a poor form of evidence!

Non-systematic review is a summary of existing knowledge that does not follow a standardised, rigorous protocol for searching, selecting or appraising studies. Randomised control trials (RCTs) is a prospective study where the participants are randomly assigned to different groups to test effectiveness of a treatment or intervention. Since they provide the most reliable evidence, RCTs are considered the gold standard for scientific research.

Delphi, from the Oracle of Delphi, an ancient Greek shrine (c. 1400 BC) where people travelled to ask prophesy from Pythia, the priestess of Apollo

13. Hand infection

A. Flexor tenosynovitis

This gentleman is displaying three out of the four Kanavel signs, thus making flexor sheath infection the most likely diagnosis. Kanavel criteria include fusiform swelling, painful flexor sheath on palpation and finger held in flexed position with pain on passive extension. It is likely that with his history of diabetes and nail biting, this flexor sheath infection has spread from a previous paronychia – infection around the nail fold. This patient will thus need urgent surgery to wash out the sheath, either with incisions made at the A1 and A4 pulley followed by catheter irrigation or via a Brunner incision. If not managed urgently, he is at risk of tendon rupture, spread of infection into palm and long-term stiffness.

A felon is an infection of the pulp space and needs to be drained to reduce the chance of compartment syndrome of the fingertip. The fingertip pulp has fibrous septa within its contents and thus creates potential for a closed space infection and neurovascular compromise. Necrotising fasciitis is an emergency caused normally by group A streptococcus. As the infection is in the deep subcutaneous tissues, it normally presents in the early stages with a mild skin rash. However, rapid progression of disease means one should be vigilant and escalate to your senior, intensive treatment unit (ITU) and plastic surgery department urgently if you consider the diagnosis. Pain out of proportion to a mild skin condition coupled with haemodynamic instability are signs one must act upon, as the patient will need extensive debridement, IV antibiotics and ITU support.

14. Mouth ulcers

D. Idiopathic aphthous ulcers

Aphthous mouth ulcers are a common idiopathic benign condition affecting up to 20% of the population. The incidence rises dramatically in the presence of inflammatory bowel disease. Although very painful, recurrent aphthous ulcers in the absence of gastrointestinal symptoms in a young person are likely to be benign. In recurrent and severe cases it may be appropriate to do blood investigations, including serum vitamin B_{12} and folate. In cases of a single prolonged ulcer of greater than 3 weeks' duration, it is prudent to take a biopsy to exclude a carcinoma. Treatment is symptomatic with topical analgesic agents.

Aphthous, from Greek *aphtha* = eruption

15. Antibiotics

E. Vancomycin – Gram-negative cover

Vancomycin is a glycopeptide antibiotic that binds D-ala-D-ala peptide sequences to prevent peptidoglycan cell wall synthesis; therefore it is active against Gram-positive but not Gram-negative bacteria (the peptidoglycan cell wall is a far more prominent and important feature in Gram-positive bacteria). Co-amoxiclav has good Gram-positive and Gram-negative cover, as well as a great deal of anaerobic cover, so is a widely used antibiotic in many scenarios; however, its broad-spectrum characteristic means it disturbs the gut flora and can predispose to *Clostridium difficile* infection. Flucloxacillin is a narrow-spectrum antibiotic with only Gram-positive cover and is often used in staphylococcal infections. Gentamicin has predominantly Gram-negative cover, although it has some Gram-positive cover as well. Metronidazole has wide anaerobic cover and is often used in surgery due to the presence of anaerobes in the bowel.

Hans Christian Joachim Gram, Danish bacteriologist (1853-1938)

Vancomycin, derived from "vanquish"

16. Pleural effusion

A. Congestive cardiac failure

Pleural effusion is characterised by the accumulation of serous fluid within the pleural space. Pleural effusion is categorised into exudative effusion (increased microvascular pressure due to disease of the pleural surface, systemic inflammation or injury in the adjacent lung) and transudative effusion (increased hydrostatic pressure or decreased osmotic pressure). Light's criteria states that pleural fluid is an exudate if one or more of the following criteria are met: (1) pleural fluid protein: serum protein ratio >0.5, (2) pleural fluid lactate dehydrogenase (LDH): serum LDH ratio >0.6 and (3) pleural fluid LDH more than two-thirds of the upper limit of normal serum LDH. The causes of exudative and transudative effusions are shown in the following table:

Exudative	Transudative
Tuberculosis	Heart failure
Pulmonary infarction	Renal failure
Pneumonia	Hypoalbuminemia.
Malignant diseases	Liver failure
Rheumatoid disease	
Systemic lupus erythematosus	
Acute pancreatitis	

17. Topical steroids

B. Dermovate

Topical steroids are categorised as mild, moderate, potent or very potent. The more potent the steroid, the more likely it is to have side effects such as skin atrophy, striae and increased risk of infection. Subsequently, the more potent the topical steroid, the less time it should be used for. Hydrocortisone is a mild steroid, Eumovate a moderate steroid, Betnovate a potent steroid, and Dermovate is a very potent steroid. Prednisolone is an oral steroid, and if the Dermovate does not get on top of the eczema, there may be a case for using systemic oral steroids – although they are not normally used in eczema and carry a greater risk of side effects when used: patients can become cushingoid, hypertensive, diabetic, immunosuppressed, osteoporotic and may develop steroid-induced psychosis.

18. Skin lesion

C. Impetigo

Itchy, red skin can be caused by various conditions, such as eczema and psoriasis, but two distinct features suggest a different diagnosis. Firstly, the spreading from a starting point, rather than patches appearing at the same time or cropping up in unrelated positions over time, suggests infection. Secondly, the honey or golden crust is a purulent discharge. Both are classic features of impetigo. Impetigo is a contagious, superficial infection caused most commonly by *Staphylococcus aureus*. The infection spreads when lesions burst to release an exudate, which spreads the bacteria outwards and leaves behind the crust. Swabs should be taken for microscopy, culture and, most importantly, sensitivities. In contained infections, topical antibiotics can be prescribed, but in more widespread disease, systemic antibiotics should be used. Antibiotics with good activity against staphylococci, such as flucloxacillin, should be used pending sensitivities. Antihistamines can be prescribed to help with itching. Underlying skin disease, such as eczema, can predispose.

Erysipelas is an infection of the superficial dermis and typically presents with erythema and a well-demarcated border. It is caused typically by group A beta-haemolytic streptococcus and seen in immunocompromised patients. Staphylococcal scalded skin syndrome typically affects neonates and follows infection with group 2 coagulase-positive staphylococci whereby a circulating epidermolytic toxin causes epidermal splitting in the granular layer, leading to peeling of the epidermis in large sections. It appears as erythema and blistering, which may exfoliate with light touch (Nikolsky sign). A focus of infection should be sought, and systemic flucloxacillin should be started along with analgesia, fluid monitoring and skin care. It normally develops over a period of hours to days and usually runs a benign course.

Impetigo, from Latin *impetere* = to assail

19. Management of Parkinson's disease

E. Postural hypotension

The fall happened soon after he stood up and involved a brief loss of consciousness, and he had an excess sympathetic discharge shortly afterwards.

It certainly sounds like an episode of postural hypotension. Standing up requires a significant degree of autonomic nervous system function to detect and react to the intravascular volume redistribution. As L-DOPA is a precursor in the synthesis of not only dopamine but also noradrenaline, excess peripheral noradrenaline and dopamine can cause widespread autonomic dysfunction, symptoms of which include nausea and postural hypotension. Hallucinations can occur with L-DOPA but are unlikely to cause a fall, and dyskinetic movements could cause a fall but don't explain the loss of consciousness. Multiple system atrophy (MSA), a Parkinson-plus syndrome, indeed includes prominent autonomic dysfunction; however, it is extremely rare and would be less likely to respond well to L-DOPA therapy (as this man has).

20. Arrhythmias

C. A form of ventricular tachycardia that can self-correct but can also lead to sudden death

Torsades de pointes is a rare form of ventricular tachycardia. If a new waveform was drawn by joining up the peaks and troughs, it would look roughly sinusoidal. The name derives from the sense that appears as if a normal electrocardiogram (ECG) were rotating in time around the isoelectric baseline (i.e. rising out of the page with positive amplitude, rotating toward the reader and falling back in with negative amplitude). The expression was first coined in 1966 by Francois Dessertenne. Torsades de pointes is significant in that it can both lower arterial blood pressure (leading to syncope) and is a precursor to ventricular fibrillation and therefore sudden death. It is often caused by drugs such as tricyclic antidepressants, amiodarone, clarithromycin and fluoroquinolones or electrolyte disturbance secondary to malnutrition and alcohol abuse. There are congenital conditions such as Romano–Ward syndrome which also predispose to long QT syndrome and torsades de pointes. It is treated with removing and correcting the trigger, intravenous magnesium and anti-arrhythmics with consideration of a pacemaker.

Torsades de pointes, from French *torsades de pointes* = twisting of the points

Francois Dessertenne, contemporary French physician

21. Back pain

C. Magnetic resonance imaging (MRI) of the whole spine

This man is presenting with advanced signs of spinal cord compression. Initially this may present with sensory deficit and weakness and progress to bladder and bowel disturbance. Spinal cord compression needs to be considered in any patient presenting with acute back pain, but a higher index of suspicion is required in patients with known malignancy, as metastases to the spine may be a cause. Spinal cord compression is an emergency that requires prompt diagnosis to prevent lasting deficit. Therefore, an urgent MRI of the whole spine is appropriate to visualise the lesion and the extent of compression. MRI is a better medium than CT scan, as it allows better visualisation of the soft tissues of the spinal cord. Treatment will depend on the cause but may include urgent referral for neurosurgery.

22. Bruising in children

A. Acute lymphoblastic leukaemia

Acute lymphoblastic leukaemia (ALL) is the most common leukaemia in children and is caused by the abnormal clonal proliferation of lymphoid pre-cursor (blast) cells that have been arrested at an early stage of development. The blast cells infiltrate the marrow and lymphoid tissue, causing pancyto-penia and lymphadenopathy, respectively. ALL is most common in child-hood with peak incidence at 3–4 years. The central nervous system can also be affected, causing headache, vomiting, meningism, cranial nerve palsies and seizure. The marrow failure and subsequent pancytopenia produce the common features of anaemia, bleeding/bruising and infection. Bone pain is another common presenting symptom. A full blood count confirms anae-mia and thrombocytopenia but demonstrates a high white cell count (due to circulating blast cells). The investigation of choice is bone marrow aspira-tion, which shows a hypercellular marrow with >20% blast cells. Lumbar puncture is often also necessary in the initial setting to detect cerebral involvement. Treatment is transfusions and antibiotics and chemotherapy. Chemotherapy is traditionally delivered in three main stages: remission induction, consolidation and maintenance, which can be for a number of years. Since patients with ALL are at high risk of neurological disease, they are often given central nervous system prophylaxis in the form of intrathecal methotrexate and radiotherapy. The prognosis of ALL is good with appro-priate treatment, and 95% of children can be expected to achieve remission.

23. Management of skin lesions

B. Oral or IV aciclovir pending ophthalmology review

This patient has shingles following human herpes virus infection. Herpes zoster is caused by the varicella zoster virus, which is responsible for chick-enpox. After an episode of chickenpox, the virus resides in dorsal root/geniculate or trigeminal ganglia and can be transported retrogradely along the sensory axons to emerge and cause herpes zoster, most commonly in a dermatomal distribution (although it can be diffuse, usually in immuno-suppressed patients). It appears most commonly along the thoracic nerves on the trunk; however, it can affect branches of the trigeminal nerve, most commonly the ophthalmic, where it can also cause conjunctivitis, keratitis or iridocyclitis. It may also affect the facial nerve and present as Ramsay

Hunt syndrome. Concurrent illness or immunosuppression can trigger zoster, and it is more common in the elderly. There are three potential phases: pre-eruptive whereby peri- and intraneural inflammation causes paraesthesia. Eruption is the demonstration of vesicular lesions, which eventually crust over after 7–10 days. Occasionally there is a chronic phase as well, which is also known as post-herpetic neuralgia. Many episodes will resolve spontaneously after around 2 weeks, so the decision to treat depends on severity. This patient has ocular involvement, and an ophthalmologist must be involved early on to decide whether the patient needs oral or IV aciclovir. This patient will also require regular eye care. Topical aciclovir or steroids are unlikely to help, and topical antibiotics are not indicated unless there is concurrent bacterial infection. Without prompt treatment, the patient has a higher chance to develop post-herpetic neuralgia, as well as visual loss.

Varicella, from Latin *variola* = spotted

Herpes, from Greek *herpein* = to crawl

Zoster, from Greek *zoster* = a belt or zone

24. Coarctation of the aorta

B. Electrocardiogram

Coarctation is a narrowing of the aorta and is more commonly seen in people diagnosed with Turner's syndrome. It typically occurs at the level of the ductus/ligament arteriosum; however, it may be pre- or post-ductal. It is a congenital deformity and may be asymptomatic or present as a child failing to thrive, palpitations, syncope or pain in the lower limbs. Coarctation of the aorta is accurately diagnosed by magnetic resonance angiography. An ECG does not normally show any diagnostic changes. Collateral vessels may be visible around the scapulae. Upper limb pulses are stronger than lower limb pulses, and this can be an indicator of coarctation in the absence of peripheral vascular disease (unlikely in a 14 year old) but only if the brachial artery assessed is proximal to the coarctation. The coarctation may reside between the right brachiocephalic artery and the left subclavian artery, leading to radial pulse asymmetry, or distal to them both, leading to radiofemoral delay. A reduced ankle–brachial pressure index may also be present. Coarctation of the aorta is often managed with surgical dilation and stenting.

25. Management of asthma

A. Add an inhaled long-acting beta-2 agonist

According to the updated joint NICE, British Thoracic Society (BTS) and Scottish Intercollegiate Guidelines Network (SIGN) guidelines of 2024, every patient with asthma should be started on both a short-acting beta-agonist and a steroid inhaler. If required, then a long-acting beta-agonist such as salmeterol could be added. One may consider increasing the dose of steroids further if asthma remains uncontrolled. The next steps in management would be the addition of leukotriene receptor antagonists followed by oral steroids. It is important to engage the patient in their own management, ensuring correct inhaler technique and a reduction in exposure to triggers such as smoking. After commencing or adjusting treatment, it is recommended that the response to treatment be reviewed every 8–12 weeks.

26. Collapse

B. Adrenal insufficiency

Hyponatraemia and hyperkalaemia in a patient presenting with postural hypotension indicates a possible diagnosis of primary adrenal insufficiency (Addison's disease). Adrenal insufficiency results in an inadequate secretion of cortisol and/or aldosterone. Features of an acute adrenal crisis include hyponatraemia, hyperkalaemia and circulatory shock with severe hypotension. There may be unexplained pyrexia, nausea and vomiting, diarrhoea and muscle cramps.

The short Synacthen test is used for the diagnosis of adrenal insufficiency. Synacthen, a synthetic adrenocorticotropic hormone (ACTH) analogue, is given to the patient and the cortisol response is noted. In normal individuals, Synacthen will stimulate the adrenal cortex to secrete cortisol. In patients with adrenal insufficiency, however, the cortex is unable to respond, and the cortisol levels remain low. A cortisol level of >550 nmol/L at 30 minutes after Synacthen administration excludes adrenal insufficiency.

If the result is positive or equivocal, the patient should have a long Synacthen test. Here cortisol is measured at 1, 4, 8 and 24 hours after Synacthen administration. In primary adrenal insufficiency (Addison's disease) the cortisol will never exceed 550 nmol/L. If the insufficiency is caused by corticotrophin-releasing hormone (CRH) or ACTH deficiency, it is termed "secondary adrenal deficiency". In secondary adrenal insufficiency, the cortisol level is likely to surpass 550 nmol/L but the response is delayed. Treatment is usually with supplementary hydrocortisone and fludrocortisone. One must also educate the patient to carry steroid cards, as it is likely the regular dose of steroids will need to be increased on admission to hospital.

27. Diagnosis of abdominal pain

E. Spontaneous bacterial peritonitis (SBP)

Patients with ascites are at risk of developing SBP, which usually presents with severe generalised abdominal pain, worsening ascites, vomiting, fever and rigors. The most common causative organisms are Gram-negative bacilli such as *Escherichia coli* and *Klebsiella* spp., which enter the systemic circulation from the intestinal lumen and colonise the ascitic fluid. SBP can lead to rapid decompensation of liver disease causing hepatic encephalopathy and death. The diagnosis is confirmed by paracentesis, which involves taking a sample of ascitic fluid from the abdomen using a needle. The aspirated ascitic fluid is analysed for white cell count, glucose and protein. In addition, the fluid should be sent to microbiology for culture and Gram staining. If the white cell count is above 250 cells/mm^3, the patient requires intravenous antibiotics (e.g. cefotaxime or ceftriaxone). Some patients also require human albumin solution to restore their intravascular fluid volume. Patients who have had a previous episode of SBP and patients who are considered to be at high risk of developing SBP should be considered for prophylactic oral antibiotics (e.g. norfloxacin or ciprofloxacin). The development of SBP corresponds to a poor long-term prognosis.

28. Investigation of stroke

A. Carotid Doppler

The carotid Doppler is unlikely to be helpful, as the infarct was clearly in the posterior circulation territory. The ECG may reveal atrial fibrillation, which is especially a possibility given his hyperthyroidism. As he is quite young for a stroke, it is important to be aware of unusual causes; a full blood count (FBC) may reveal polycythaemia (he is a smoker in his 50s) or an abnormal platelet reading, and the ESR may be elevated if there is a vasculitic process behind the infarct – he has a background of autoimmune disease. Magnetic resonance angiography (MRA) will show if there is an obvious site of posterior circulation occlusion, and in the absence of any obvious reason, this may be helpful in guiding further investigation and management, e.g. intravenous angiography +/– stenting for vertebral artery dissection.

29. Diagnosis of cough

C. Sarcoidosis

Sarcoidosis is a multisystem granulomatous disease of unknown cause. It commonly affects adults aged 20–40 years old. Afro-Caribbean individuals are affected more frequently and more severely than Caucasians, particularly in terms of extrathoracic disease. Around 20–40% of patients are asymptomatic, and it is discovered incidentally on chest X-ray. Of patients with a pulmonary component of sarcoidosis, 90% have an abnormal chest X-ray with bilateral hilar lymphadenopathy with or without pulmonary infiltrates or fibrosis. Symptoms include dry cough, progressive dyspnoea, reduced exercise tolerance and chest pain. Other features include erythema nodosum (painful, purple, tender lesions on the shins); lupus pernio (sarcoidosis lesions on the skin); arthralgia; and lymphadenopathy. Sarcoidosis tissue can activate vitamin D and cause hypercalcaemia.

Serum calcium and angiotensin-converting enzyme (ACE) levels are elevated, and the tuberculin test is negative. The diagnosis of sarcoidosis is confirmed by biopsy and histology (showing non-caseating granulomas). The Kveim–Siltzbach test – where a sample of splenic tissue is injected into the skin in order to try and produce granulation tissue – is no longer done. Sarcoidosis is staged according to chest X-ray findings as follows:

Stage 1: Bilateral hilar lymphadenopathy

Stage 2: Bilateral hilar lymphadenopathy and lung involvement

Stage 3: Lung involvement only

Stage 4: Lung fibrosis

Treatment is with steroids and immunosuppressants.

Sarcoidosis, from Greek *sark* = flesh (+ -oid) i.e. flesh-like, describing the granulomatous deposition seen in the disease

Morton Ansgar Kveim, Norwegian pathologist (1892-1966)

Louis Siltzbach, American physician (1906-1980)

30. Diagnosis of multiple sclerosis

B. Oligoclonal bands on electrophoresis

Whilst there is sometimes a rise in lymphocytes, this is both mild and rare, and given the pathology, you might not expect to see red blood cells in the cerebrospinal fluid, which is backed up by observation. The protein level can be elevated, but this is rather non-specific. Whilst no single specific antigen has been identified in multiple sclerosis (MS), antibodies to various myelinating cell-associated proteins have been found in patients with MS, myelin basic protein among them. However, testing for this autoantibody alone would not be sensitive enough. Oligoclonal bands on electrophoresis are found in 50–60% of patients after the first attack and up to 95% of patients with established disease. Whilst this isn't entirely MS specific, being found in chronic meningitis, neurosarcoidosis and rare infectious nervous system diseases, they persist indefinitely in MS, unlike the other disorders, and when combined with an appropriate clinical picture, are highly suggestive of multiple sclerosis.

31. Investigation of abdominal pain

D. Hepatic vein Doppler ultrasound scan (USS)

Sudden-onset ascites with tender hepatomegaly in the absence of jaundice should hold a high degree of suspicion for Budd–Chiari syndrome. This syndrome describes the effects of hepatic vein outflow obstruction, commonly by thrombosis or malignant obstruction. Risk factors include malignancy, thrombophilias such as polycythaemia vera, trauma and the oral contraceptive pill. This can present either acutely or chronically. Diagnosis is made by Doppler scanning of the hepatic vein or venography. A similar clinical picture is produced by right-sided heart failure, constrictive peri-carditis and inferior vena cava obstruction, which should also be excluded during your investigations. Treatment depends on the cause but may involve heparin, thrombolysis and liver transplant. Polycythaemia vera is typically caused by a *JAK2* mutation leading to bone marrow proliferation of red blood cells, in turn leading to an increased clotting potential.

George Budd , English physician (1808-1882)

Hans Chiari , Austrian pathologist (1851-1916)

32. Diagnosis of cough

D. Tuberculosis

Tuberculosis (TB) is the most common infection in the world, with a greater risk in developing countries, human immunodeficiency virus (HIV) infec-tion and malnutrition. Although the incidence of TB in northwestern Europe and North America has declined in the latter half of the twentieth century, case rates have increased over the past 10 years secondary to immi-gration, the spread of HIV/AIDS and the neglect of TB control programmes.

TB is caused by the Gram-positive organism *Mycobacterium tuber-culosis*, although some cases are caused by *Mycobacterium bovis* and *Mycobacterium africanum*. Primary TB infection occurs through droplet infection and leads to the development of the primary lung lesion (a focus of TB organisms surrounded by macrophages, known as the Ghon focus). This may be associated with enlarged hilar lymph nodes (Ghon complex) but is often asymptomatic. The pathology of TB is caseating granulomas. Spontaneous healing occurs in 90% of primary lesions, although a severe, disseminated infection occurs in 10% (miliary TB – seen as 1- to 2-mm fine lesions through the lung fields on X-ray). Reinfection or reactivation of TB results in post-primary disease. Post-primary pulmonary TB presents with a subacute illness with cough, haemoptysis, dyspnoea, fever, night sweats and anorexia. A chest X-ray shows lesions in the upper lobes. Features of extrapulmonary TB include painless lymphadenopathy, constrictive peri-carditis, ascites, spinal disease, septic arthritis and kidney infection.

The diagnosis of TB can be made by sputum staining (using Ziehl–Neelsen stain) and culture (on Lowenstein–Jensen media; this can take up to 6 weeks). The bacille Calmette–Guerin (bCG) vaccine is made of attenuated *M. bovis* and provides some protection. Skin tuberculin testing can be used to screen for TB. There are two types: the Heaf test (a multipuncture method that is read after 5 days and is positive if there is ring-shaped induration) and the Mantoux test (an intradermal tuberculin injection that is read at 3 days and is positive when induration is >5 mm). False negatives to tubercu-lin screening are seen with severe TB, HIV, malnutrition, malignancy and sarcoidosis and in people taking immunosuppressants.

Drug treatment of TB is with 6 months of anti-tuberculous therapy (e.g. rifampicin, isoniazid, pyrazinamide and ethambutol for 4 months followed by just rifampicin and isoniazid for 2 months). Ethambutol can be omitted if drug resistance is unlikely (e.g. in white HIV-negative patients). Treatment is given for 12 months for central nervous system disease. Multidrug-resistant TB (MDRTB) is defined as TB infection that is resistant to rifampicin and isoniazid. MRDTB is treated with five drugs for 24 months (including clarithromycin and streptomycin). Drugs are given as a single daily dose before breakfast.

The side effects of the commonly used anti-tuberculous drugs are as follows:

- Rifampicin: Orange urine, purple tears, hepatitis, induced liver enzymes
- Isoniazid: Hepatitis, peripheral neuropathy
- Pyrazinamide: Hepatitis, photosensitivity, gout
- Ethambutol: Optic neuritis
- Streptomycin: Ototoxic, nephrotoxic

Anton Ghon, Austrian pathologist (1866-1936)

Miliary, from Latin *miliarius* = grain seeds

33. Diagnosis of tuberculosis

D. Perihilar ground-glass changes

A cavitating lesion is not the most common appearance of tuberculosis on chest X-ray, but it could represent a tuberculoma; it could also be a tumour, abscess or granuloma. Lobar consolidation can be seen and has a differential of bacterial pneumonia (although the symptoms and their length differentiate this). The diffuse, small opacifications are consistent with miliary tuberculosis, which indicates blood-borne dissemination and typically presents more acutely, often with involvement of other organs. Tuberculosis can cause pleural effusions; however, the perihilar ground-glass change does not suggest this. Hilar lymphadenopathy can be seen in tuberculosis. Finally, tuberculosis is diagnosed when the mycobacteria are seen, and multiple sputum samples should be sent for staining and culture. The absence of classical X-ray changes does not rule it out.

34. Thrombocytopenia

D. Heparin-induced thrombocytopenia (HIT)

Thrombocytopenia can be induced by a number of drugs. Low-molecular-weight heparin (LMWH) is commonly prescribed in hospital for the prevention and treatment of deep vein thrombosis and pulmonary embolism. Side effects of heparin on platelets are a relatively common idiosyncratic reaction, although there is a markedly reduced incidence when using LMWH compared to intravenous unfractionated heparin. In HIT, the platelet count reduces around 5–14 days after the initial exposure. There are two types:

1. Type 1 HIT is a non-immune transient asymptomatic thrombocytopenia that is seen in up to 10% of patients given heparin. Platelet levels usually remain above 80×10^9/mL, and no treatment is required. The platelet count improves spontaneously even when heparin is continued.
2. Type 2 HIT is a rare but serious condition that may result in multiorgan failure and death secondary to an autoimmune process. It is caused by an immune reaction against the complex of heparin and platelet factor 4.

These complexes are removed from the circulation, resulting in thrombocytopenia. However, in doing so, the release of platelet factor 4 into the circulation causes the activation of the remaining platelets. This leads to the situation of coexistent thrombocytopenia and thrombosis (arterial and venous). Type 2 HIT is seen in approximately 3–5% of patients who are prescribed unfractionated heparin but is much less common with LMWH. If type 2 HIT is suspected, heparin must be stopped immediately and an alternative treatment instigated. Thrombolytic agents such as streptokinase may be needed to treat significant thrombosis.

Evans syndrome is an autoimmune disease against red cells and platelets, resulting in an autoimmune haemolytic anaemia and thrombocytopenia.

35. Meningitis

C. Pneumococcal meningitis

The sudden onset and severe nature with sepsis preclude viral meningitis. There seems to be no overt risk of immunocompromise (homelessness, promiscuity or intravenous drug use), and the onset was acute, thus making tubercular meningitis unlikely. The lack of likely immunocompromise, age below 50 years and lack of cranial nerve involvement all point away from *Listeria* meningitis. Given the alcoholism and recent chest infection, pneumococcal meningitis seems quite likely and carries a worse prognosis than meningococcal meningitis – a 20% mortality rather than 10% in meningococcal disease. His low GCS and sepsis (fever, tachycardia and low blood pressure) are also bad signs, and this man may require intensive care unit (ITU) admission. At this point in the assessment one should focus on resuscitation, primarily ensuring an ABCDE approach is commenced with IV fluid resuscitation and antibiotics started. Ideally, blood cultures should be sent prior to starting antibiotics. A lumbar puncture will be performed and is likely to provide the causative organism before targeted therapy can be begun.

Meningitis, from Greek *menix* = membrane

36. Electrocardiogram

A. Hyperkalaemia

The T-wave on an ECG denotes the repolarisation of the myocardium after systole. In the context of a patient presenting with chest pain, an inverted T-wave is a sign of myocardial infarction (also indicated by ST elevation/depression and the development of Q-waves). A similar process, to a lesser degree, occurs in myocardial ischaemia. Left ventricular hypertrophy and left bundle branch block change the nature of ventricular myocardial repolarisation and hence may also invert the T-wave. Hyperkalaemia will increase the rate of repolarisation that leads to a peaked or "tented" T-wave rather than an inverted one. The accompanying P-wave may reduce and the QRS complex may broaden. Hyperkalaemia, commonly caused by angiotensin-converting enzyme inhibitors (ACEis), potassium sparing diuretics, acute renal failure and blood transfusions, is potentially serious and may lead to asystole or ventricular fibrillation. Hypokalaemia may flatten or invert the T-wave and yield subtle U-waves (downward deflections) after the T-wave. Hypokalaemia may lead to cardiac arrhythmias, constipation and fatigue and is commonly caused by diuretics and diarrhoea. Any abnormality of potassium should be treated seriously with appropriate reversal.

37. Diarrhoea

E. Overflow diarrhoea

Constipation is common and can be a debilitating condition in the elderly population. It can present with pain and discomfort and is more common in people who are immobile for long periods of time or on multiple analgesics. Spurious diarrhoea such as described can occur as watery stool manages to escape around the impacted faeces, often giving a mixed picture of diarrhoea on the background of constipation. Treatment for constipation begins with lifestyle, increasing the amount of fluid drunk, encouraging mobilisation where possible and withholding or changing constipating drugs such as opiates. Pharmacological treatments include osmotic laxatives such as lactulose, which draw water into the stool; a bulk-forming laxative such as bran; and stimulant laxatives such as Movicol or glycerine suppositories. This gentleman will require multidisciplinary care involving the geriatrician and physical and occupational therapist coupled with regular encouragement by the nursing home staff.

38. Management of epilepsy

D. Valproate may cause gum hypertrophy

Even when medicated, it is a Driver and Vehicle Licensing Agency (DVLA) regulation that patients abstain from driving for 1 year after their last seizure, unless they have had seizures only in their sleep for the last 3 years. Whilst the patient is under 25 years, the focal nature of the attack onset is an indication for a CT/MRI to look for a structural cause, e.g. tumour or arteriovenous malformation. Valproate can cause hair loss, thrombocytopenia and hepatitis, but gum hypertrophy is not a common side effect – it is a side effect of phenytoin.

39. Diagnosis of HIV-related illness

A. Bronchoalveolar lavage

Pneumocystis pneumonia is the most common AIDS-defining illness, caused by the fungus *Pneumocystis jiroveci* (previously known as *Pneumocystis carinii*). Patients present with a dry cough, fever, shortness of breath, weight loss and night sweats.

Bronchoalveolar lavage involves bronchoscopy and thus is quite invasive, but it is highly sensitive and 90% specific (95% with biopsy). Radiological changes can be conspicuously absent early on, but a perihilar ground-glass pattern of change can be found. Sputum cytology on sputum obtained by hypertonic saline nebuliser induction is specific although less sensitive than bronchoalveolar lavage – as low as 30% sensitive. Hypoxaemia on the arterial blood gas is a non-specific finding. The other advantage of bronchoalveolar lavage is that it will be specific in the diagnosis of other HIV-related pulmonary diseases such as tuberculosis.

Treatment is with co-trimoxazole (trimethoprim and sulphamethoxazole). Patients with HIV who have a low CD4 count (<200/µL) receive prophylaxis for *Pneumocystis* (e.g. co-trimoxazole or dapsone).

40. Tiredness

E. Vitamin B$_{12}$ deficiency

This pattern of symptoms reflects the complications of vitamin B$_{12}$ deficiency: a macrocytic anaemia, glossitis and peripheral neuropathy. Vitamin B$_{12}$ is an essential water-soluble vitamin required for DNA synthesis and red blood cell production. It is absorbed in the terminal ileum only after binding intrinsic factor, which is secreted by gastric parietal cells. The liver can store approximately 1 mg of vitamin B$_{12}$, sufficient for 3–4 years; hence B$_{12}$ deficiency takes years to manifest. The main causes of vitamin B$_{12}$ deficiency are pernicious anaemia (most common in the UK), poor dietary intake (vegans) and malabsorption secondary to disease of the terminal ileum. Pernicious anaemia describes the autoimmune loss of parietal cells and/or intrinsic factor, thus preventing the absorption of vitamin B$_{12}$. It is most common in women over 60 years. Around 90% of patients demonstrate anti-parietal antibodies (but some normal women also have it), and 60% are found to have anti-intrinsic factor antibody (which is a more specific marker).

Patients with bowel pathology, such as Crohn's disease, have normal levels of intrinsic factor but cannot absorb the B_{12}-intrinsic factor complex due to disease of the terminal ileum. Although most patents with pernicious anaemia complain of lethargy and general malaise, specific features of vitamin B_{12} deficiency include peripheral neuropathy, smooth tongue, angular stomatitis, depression, dementia and subacute degeneration of the spinal cord. Subacute degeneration of the spinal cord predominately affects the posterior columns and presents as subtle ataxia, reduced proprioception and peripheral neuropathy. When suspected, an MRI of the spine will aid the diagnosis.

The blood film is likely to show a macrocytic (↑ mean corpuscular volume [MCV]), megaloblastic anaemia with hypersegmented neutrophil nuclei (six or more lobes). In addition, serum vitamin B_{12} levels are low and ferritin levels are normal, reflecting normal iron stores. The two-part Schilling test distinguishes pernicious anaemia from intestinal causes of B_{12} deficiency. Treatment is with hydroxocobalamin (an intramuscular preparation of vitamin B_{12}), which is given as a 1-mg dose every other day until the blood film and symptoms improve, followed by 1-mg injections every 3 months.

As a side note, when investigating patients for anaemia, if folate deficiency is discovered, one must check B_{12} levels, as correcting folate before B_{12} levels will mask B_{12} deficiency and may lead to worsening of neurological function.

The term "megaloblast" describes an abnormally large, nucleated erythrocyte precursor found in people deficient in B_{12} or folate

41. Management of acne

A. It commonly leads to hearing loss

Isotretinoin is a vitamin A analogue that markedly reduces the production of sebum. Increased sebum production is believed to contribute to the pathogenesis of acne vulgaris, as hair follicles blocked off with hyperkeratosis, which subsequently have raised sebum production within, become comedones, and it is here that the conditions are rife for *Proprionibacterium acnes* to proliferate and induce an inflammatory response. When other therapies have failed, lesions are severe, scarring is beginning to form, or a patient is psychologically affected, systemic isotretinoin can be used. This can lead to complete clearance in 90% of patients. Hearing loss is a very rare side effect. Dry lips are an extremely common side effect. Other skin areas can also become very dry – this is the mode of action of the drug, so the patient must attempt to put up with it as much as possible rather than cover the dry skin in thick moisturisers. Isotretinoin is highly teratogenic, and therefore with female patients of reproductive age, a frank discussion should be held regarding contraception. Hyperlipidaemia and raised liver function tests are common and are therefore monitored during treatment. Any derangement of these tests often resolves after termination of therapy.

There are some reports of an increased incidence of depression amongst patients taking isotretinoin, although these are not consistently reproduced, and the return of someone's skin to a normal appearance can often ameliorate depression rather than cause it. Patients should be warned that there is a concern that some patients might become depressed when on isotretinoin and to be vigilant for this, but not that most people feel depressed, as this is untrue.

One should ensure to advise the patient not to over-clean her face – twice daily is sufficient. She should also ensure to maintain a healthy diet and lifestyle.

Acne, from Latin *acne* = eruption

42. Epigastric pain

E. Upper gastrointestinal (GI) endoscopy

Both gastric and oesophageal cancer can have a devastating prognosis, as they generally present late. Risk factors are similar and include increasing age, smoking, alcohol, gastritis/oesophagitis and Barrett's oesophagus. Signs and symptoms are often vague, with epigastric pain/retrosternal pain, progressive dysphagia and/or dyspepsia with weight loss and indication for endoscopy. Endoscopy is the investigation of choice, as it allows for a tissue diagnosis and histology, with CT being a supplementary study to determine stage and metastases. One must be cautious to increase the anti-reflux medication prior to thorough investigation, as it may lead to further delays in treatment and thus worsen the overall prognosis.

43. Skin loss

C. Toxic epidermal necrolysis

This woman is suffering from toxic epidermal necrolysis (TEN), a rare condition which typically follows initiation of a medication, including certain antibiotics, allopurinol and antiepileptics. The pathogenesis is not known, but it is believed to be either due to an over-activation of T cells or over-expression of apoptotic pathways, which leads to the clinical picture. Patients often present with progressive skin loss involving >30% of the body surface area, distinguishing it from Stevens–Johnson syndrome (SJS; <10%). Blistering occurs as the epidermis peels from the dermis with a collection of fluid between the two layers. One may see Nikolsky's sign – a peeling of skin with light touch. Patients are at risk of dehydration, sepsis and multiorgan failure and should be managed ideally in an ICU burn centre, as they often require multiorgan support including ventilation, vasopressors and renal replacement therapy. Regular analgesia and dressing changes will be required. The offending medication should be discontinued, with further antibiotics, steroids and immunoglobulin therapy considered. The SCORTEN criteria provide prognostic value.

44. Management of DKA

A. Intravenous insulin at a dose of 0.1 units/kg/hour until blood glucose <14 mmol/L and then switch to 0.05 units/kg/hour

To diagnose DKA all three of the following must be met: capillary blood glucose above 11 mmol/L and capillary ketones above 3 mmol/L or urine ketones ++ or more and venous pH less than 7.3 and/or bicarbonate less than 15 mmol/L. According to the Joint British Diabetes Societies for Inpatient Care, patients in DKA should receive urgent treatment with crystalloid fluids (usually 0.9% saline), electrolyte replacement and intravenous insulin. Regular monitoring is required, as the dose of insulin must be changed according to the blood glucose levels. In particular, if blood glucose is ≥14, insulin should be administered at a dose of 0.1 units/kg/hour until blood glucose <14 mmol/L, at which point this must be switched to 0.05 units/kg/hour.

45. Renal transplantation

B. High-pressure urinary tract, e.g. posterior urethral valves

Active or chronic infection is a contraindication, as the required immunosuppression could lead to extreme worsening of infection and transplant failure. Malignancy not only could spread to the transplant but could become worse with immunosuppression, and the patient is also likely to have a shortened life expectancy. If the iliac vessels are stenosed, the transplanted kidney is unlikely to be perfused well enough to function properly (given that the blood supply to the transplant comes from the iliac vessels). Severe ischaemic heart disease is a contraindication to renal transplantation.

Posterior urethral valves can affect male newborns and can be mild or severe in their obstruction of the urinary tract. Without timely intervention, the urinary tract (including the bladder) can become high pressure and the kidneys can fail. Transplanting a new kidney onto a high-pressure tract is likely to accelerate failure of the transplant. This needn't prevent transplant, and, if it is a severe problem, an ileal conduit or neobladder can be formed as an alternative to the high-pressure tract.

46. Thrombolysis in stroke

C. 2 hours post-onset, BP 160/95 mmHg, GCS 15, MRI shows infarct

Thrombolysis has been proven to decrease death and severe disability if given within 3 hours of the onset of symptoms in ischaemic stroke. Some centres have started treating within 6 hours of symptom onset, so the patient who presented 7 hours after onset is ineligible. Blood pressure above

180/110 mmHg conveys too high a risk of haemorrhage post thrombolysis. Thrombolysis is obviously contraindicated by anything on a brain scan suggesting haemorrhage. A low Glasgow Coma Score also precludes thrombolytic treatment, which leaves patient C.

47. Diagnosis of chest pain

A. Acute pericarditis

The acute pericarditis, secondary to a viral infection, has caused these symptoms. In addition, heart sounds may be soft, indicating a pericardial effusion is underway. A chest X-ray could confirm this by demonstrating a globular heart. Cardiac tamponade is usually caused by a penetrating wound to the heart, causing haemorrhage into the pericardium. As the fibrous pericardium is inelastic, the bleed reduces the room into which the diastolic heart can expand and this, in turn, reduces cardiac output and may well be fatal. It can be treated by puncturing the pericardium with a large-bore needle to allow relief of the pressure (pericardiocentesis). Whilst the needle is inserted, it should be kept in contact with an ECG lead; the live trace will jump when the needle reaches the myocardium (too far). Once tamponade has been ruled out, she can be managed with NSAIDs and colchicine. Pulmonary embolus is a possible diagnosis for this woman but is less likely given the ECG findings.

48. Management of oliguria

B. Flush the catheter with 50 mL warm saline and then aspirate

The problem that seems to have occurred here, and is quick and easy to diagnose, is that blood clots are being retained and blocking the end of the catheter (clot retention). Flushing the catheter with some warm saline and then aspirating may dislodge the clot and allow some urine and smaller clots to pass through the catheter. It may also allow the larger clot to pass through or disrupt it and allow its fragments to pass through. If this needs to be done repeatedly, a large-bore three-way catheter (with a separate channel for irrigation) can be inserted. Removing the catheter alone is unlikely to resolve the fact that clots are blocking the urinary tract. Insertion of a suprapubic catheter seems unnecessary at this stage and is associated with a high morbidity due to potential perforation of the bowel, and severe urinary tract infections can occur. Requesting a CT KUB is not required at this stage, and if any imaging is desired a USS will demonstrate hydroureter/hydronephrosis. Due to the patient's co-morbidities, particularly dementia, he may indeed be slightly dry, but clinically this is not the most likely cause of the renal impairment. A fluid challenge could be given if an obstructive uropathy can be ruled out to see if hypovolaemia was indeed the cause.

E. **Subdural haematoma**

The first thing to note is that it is possible that the low GCS and confusion could be due to something separate, e.g. overuse of opioids and an otherwise asymptomatic urinary tract infection (UTI) – but opioid use is likely to have been highest on admission, with the pain from the injury subsequently decreasing. Action should be taken to rule out such possibilities, but as the defects have all started together, an intracranial cause would be the most worrying explanation, and an intracranial lesion must be considered. Whilst meningitis can give focal neurological defects and a decreased GCS, the stable observations; lack of a temperature; and lack of reported headache, neck stiffness or photophobia make this unlikely. A lacunar infarct can present as a pure motor weakness with no other focal defect. However, this is likely to come on acutely with decreased reflexes and is unlikely to be accompanied with a drop in GCS. Subarachnoid haemorrhage can present with a drop in GCS and focal neurology but more commonly presents with unconsciousness, seizures or thunderclap headache with meningism, which are all absent. There is no reason in the question why a subarachnoid haemorrhage would cause deficits to appear at this stage. Strokes do not usually cause a drop in GCS, although a large intracerebral haemorrhage could by mass effect; however, the neurology in the patient is subacute, mild and limited.

This patient is an elderly woman who could have possibly sustained a head injury and may be an alcoholic – these factors put her at risk of a subdural haemorrhage. Subdural haemorrhage commonly presents with a subacute development of impaired GCS and focal neurology. Due to the nature of a bleeding bridging vein, the primary insult may have been related to this admission or a prior fall. Elderly and alcohol-dependant patients are at risk due to cerebral atrophy. The reduced GCS is concerning, as it may indicate an increased intracranial pressure with potential mid-line shift and compression of the medulla. An urgent computed tomography (CT) scan of the head is indicated and the result discussed with the neurosurgeons.

The Monro–Kellie doctrine recognises the skull to be a fixed entity with three internal components – blood, cerebrospinal fluid (CSF) and cerebral tissue. A rise in intracranial pressure eventually leads to a reduced cerebral perfusion pressure. With a reduction in cerebral perfusion pressure one will see a fall in GCS. The body tries to reduce intracranial pressure by limiting the volume of intracranial components individually. Cerebral tissue is the last to be sacrificed in a process termed coning.

Get ahead! Medicine

50. Thyrotoxicosis

A. Graves' disease

This is a typical picture of a person who has thyrotoxicosis in which the most common symptoms are weight loss with a normal or increased appetite, heat intolerance, palpitations, tremor and irritability. In all causes of thyrotoxicosis, the patient would present with lid lag and lid retraction. Graves' disease is the only cause of other ophthalmological symptoms such as periorbital oedema, conjunctival irritation, exophthalmos and diplopia.

Graves' disease is the most common cause of hyperthyroidism. It is an autoimmune disease in which circulating IgG immunoglobulins incite the thyroid-stimulating hormone (TSH) receptors of the thyroid gland, causing the release of thyroxine into the circulation. Autoantibodies are also directed against retro-orbital structures causing proptosis, ophthalmoplegia and peri-orbital oedema. Treatment is typically with carbimazole, radio-iodine and/or thyroidectomy.

Robert James Graves, Irish physician (1797-1853)

Practice paper 3: Questions

1. Acute coronary syndrome

A 55-year-old man has presented to the medical admissions unit with chest pain. You have diagnosed acute coronary syndrome (ACS) and are about to write up his drug chart.

Your most suitable prescription would be:

A 75 mg aspirin, 75 mg clopidogrel, heparin with glyceryl trinitrite (GTN) spray and morphine PRN

B 75 mg aspirin, 300 mg clopidogrel, heparin and beta-blocker with GTN spray and morphine PRN

C 300 mg aspirin, 300 mg clopidogrel, oxygen (if hypoxic), heparin, beta-blocker, ACEi, with GTN spray morphine and metoclopramide PRN

D 300 mg aspirin, 300 mg clopidogrel, oxygen, heparin and beta-blocker with GTN spray and morphine PRN

E 300 mg aspirin, heparin and beta-blocker with GTN spray and morphine PRN

2. Haematuria

A 32-year-old man presents to the GP 4 days after an episode of painless haematuria 2 weeks following a sore throat. He says he now feels he is producing less urine than usual and that it is brown. He denies any weight loss or fatigue and has no family history of urological malignancy. On examination, he has a blood pressure of 155/90 mmHg, +++ blood on urine dipstick and blood tests reveal a creatinine of 170 μmol/L and normal electrolytes.

What is the clinical picture most consistent with?

A Acute tubular necrosis
B Nephritic syndrome
C Nephrotic syndrome
D Renal calculi
E Transitional cell carcinoma of the bladder

DOI: 10.1201/9781003648222-5

3. Heart failure

In the treatment of heart failure with atrial fibrillation, which of the following statements about digoxin is FALSE?

A ACE inhibitors and beta-blockers are more effective at extending survival
B Digoxin has a secondary vagal effect that slows the heart rate
C Digoxin has a narrow therapeutic index
D Digoxin is obtained from foxgloves
E Digoxin is primarily a positive chronotropic drug

4. Hodgkin's lymphoma

A 32-year-old man is diagnosed with Hodgkin's lymphoma following a recent history of weight loss and night sweats. Computed tomography (CT) staging scan shows disease in the mediastinum bilaterally and some abdominal lymphadenopathy, including the spleen, but no evidence of disease in extra-nodal sites.

What is his stage of disease?

A Stage IIA
B Stage IIB
C Stage IIIA
D Stage IIIB
E Stage IVB

5. Management of psoriasis

A 35-year-old woman with a 1-year history of plaque psoriasis is having difficulty with management. Along with emollients, she has tried tar and dithranol, which she did not get on well with (due to the smell and burning, respectively) and has been using a combination of vitamin D analogues and Betnovate, a potent topical steroid. She has difficulty finding time with her lifestyle to apply the creams often enough, and as a result the lesions have become more widespread, and she is now extremely concerned about her appearance, both in the workplace and at her sister's wedding, which is coming up soon.

Which of the following would be the best treatment to try next?

A Ciclosporin
B Infliximab
C Methotrexate
D Prednisolone
E Ultraviolet therapy

6. Subarachnoid haemorrhage

Which of the following statements about subarachnoid haemorrhage is NOT true?

A Focal weakness may ensue
B Lumbar puncture (LP) immediately on admission is likely to show xanthochromia
C Subarachnoid haemorrhage may present as a new onset of seizures
D Subarachnoid haemorrhages may be provoked by exertion or coitus
E Unenhanced CT within 6 hours is >97% sensitive

7. Overdose and antidotes

A 32-year-old woman presents to the emergency department having reportedly taken a large dose of heroin. She is unresponsive, has small pupils and has a respiratory rate of 6 breaths/min.

Which of the following should be administered?

A Atropine
B Ethanol
C Flumazenil
D N-acetylcysteine
E Naloxone

8. Pneumonia

A 44-year-old man presents to the emergency department with a 3-day history of shortness of breath and a productive cough. His temperature is 38.2°C, pulse rate 90 bpm, blood pressure 130/86 mmHg, respiratory rate 24/min and saturations 94% on room air. Blood results include white cell count of 13.5×10^6/L, CRP 45 mmol/L, Na^+ 136 mmol/L, K^+ 4.3 mmol/L, urea 9.2 mmol/L and creatinine 110 µmol/L. On examination, he appears alert with dull sounds on percussion over the right lower lobe. A chest X-ray confirms a right lower lung lobe consolidation.

What is the most appropriate management?

A Admission into hospital with empirical antibiotic treatment
B Admission into hospital for nebulised salbutamol and empirical antibiotic treatment
C Admission into intensive care unit
D Home with inhaled salbutamol when clinically stable
E Home with empirical antibiotic treatment when clinically stable

9. Murmur

A 68-year-old obese woman is not coping at home and presents to the emergency department following a fall. On examination, she has a weak, regular pulse and an ejection systolic murmur. You try to lean her forward but she gets flustered and complains of a sore back and shortness of breath. A neurological examination is unremarkable, and her haemoglobin level is 13.2 g/dL.

What is most likely wrong with her?

A Aortic stenosis
B Atrial fibrillation
C Cerebrovascular accident

D Gastrointestinal bleed
E Mitral regurgitation

10. Skin lesions

A 70-year-old man presents with multiple widespread tense blisters measuring between 0.5 and 5 cm in diameter. They are localised mainly to the arms and legs, with some lesions on the chest. They appeared over weeks, preceded by itchy urticarial lesions. A few lesions have burst and have left not much behind. There is a history of osteoarthritis of the knees for which he takes diclofenac, and he has not changed any medication in the past year. A subsequent biopsy of a bulla shows splitting at the dermo-epidermal junction.

What is the diagnosis?

A Insect bites
B Pemphigoid
C Pemphigus

D Stevens–Johnson syndrome
E Toxic epidermal necrolysis

11. Antibiotics

Which of the following antibiotic and side effect pairings is FALSE?

A Ceftriaxone and tendon rupture
B Co-amoxiclav and cholestatic jaundice
C Erythromycin and diarrhoea
D Gentamicin and nephrotoxicity
E Nitrofurantoin and pulmonary fibrosis

12. Scoring systems

Which of the following scoring systems should be used to assess a patient's risk of developing a pressure score?

A Breslow score
B Confusion, urea, respiratory rate, blood pressure, age (CURB) score
C Ranson's criteria
D Rockall score
E Waterlow score

13. Investigation of headache

A 78-year-old woman who has recently been feeling under the weather and losing some weight develops a severe, left-sided headache with jaw pain on eating. She also complains of blurred vision on the left side.

Which of the following investigations is needed to give a definitive diagnosis?

A Computed tomography (CT) of the head
B Erythrocyte sedimentation rate (ESR)
C Magnetic resonance imaging (MRI) of the head
D Temporal artery biopsy
E Ultrasound of the temporal arteries

14. Acutely swollen leg

A 22-year-old woman has attended accident and emergency with a painful left knee after colliding with another skier at a dry ski slope. Her knee is swollen, particularly in the infra-patella region, and tender to touch. It is a closed injury. Her X-ray shows she has a tibial plateau fracture associated with lipohaemathrosis with no significant displacement or dislocation. She is neurovascularly intact distally at the time of your assessment. You have informed the orthopaedic team; however, they are busy and say it may be a couple of hours before they can see her. You apply a knee brace and provide analgesia awaiting orthopaedic review. You are informed an hour later by the nurse in accident and emergency that her pain is not settling despite morphine. On re-examination you note blistering to her skin overlying the tibia, erythema, intense swelling of the leg and increasing pain on passive movement of the toes. What is your diagnosis?

A Compartment syndrome
B Acute ischaemic limb
C Poorly controlled pain
D Cellulitis
E Deep vein thrombosis

15. Management of skin lesions

An 81-year-old retired farmer presents with a 1.5-cm raised lesion on his left temple that has slowly grown over the past year and occasionally bleeds. He has had a basal cell carcinoma removed from his right temple previously, and he has had cryotherapy for actinic keratoses on his temples and head several times at his GP surgery. On examination, the lesion has a rolled edge and is translucent with telangiectasia.

Which of the following treatment options is NOT recommended for this lesion?

A Chemotherapy
B Excision
C Mohs micrographic surgery
D Radiotherapy
E Topical 5-fluorouracil

16. Fatigue

A 35-year-old man presents to the GP with increasing fatigue for 3 months. He finds himself waking up choking a few times at night. He was told by his partner that he snores quite loudly most nights. He denies any weight loss. He smokes 30 cigarettes a day, drinks 2 pints of beer every night and has a body mass index of 32 kg/m².

What is the most likely differential diagnosis?

A Central sleep apnoea
B Chronic fatigue syndrome
C Idiopathic hypersomnolence
D Narcolepsy
E Obstructive sleep apnoea

17. Arterial blood gases

A 73-year-old man has been admitted with severe sepsis and acute renal failure secondary to a urinary tract infection. He has been treated with intravenous antibiotics and fluid resuscitation, but the following day you are called to see him, as he is worse. He looks extremely unwell. His airway is patent, and he has laboured breathing at a rate of 22 breaths/min. His saturations are 98% on air, and his chest sounds clear. His pulse is 120 bpm and blood pressure is 85/55 mmHg. His capillary refill rate is 4 seconds. His urine output has been 40 mL in the last 5 hours. You see from his blood tests that his creatinine level has increased slightly. You take an arterial blood gas reading.

Which of the following is the most likely result?

A pH 7.22, pO_2 8, pCO_2 8.3, HCO_3^- 24
B pH 7.22, pO_2 18, pCO_2 2.3, HCO_3^- 10
C pH 7.22, pO_2 18, pCO_2 8.3, HCO_3^- 10
D pH 7.40, pO_2 8, pCO_2 8.3, HCO_3^- 38
E pH 7.51, pO_2 18, pCO_2 2.3, HCO_3^- 24

18. Shortness of breath

A 65-year-old man presents to the GP with chest pain, increasing shortness of breath and weight loss. He describes the pain as dull and worse on inhalation. He notices that he has lost 1 stone in 3 weeks. He has never smoked and has no other significant past medical history. He used to work in a shipyard. Observations include temperature 36.8°C, pulse rate 80 bpm, blood pressure 140/95 mmHg and respiratory rate 18/min. On examination, there is dullness to percussion over the left lower lung zone.

What is the most likely diagnosis?

A Bronchocarcinoma
B Mesothelioma
C Pneumoconiosis
D Pulmonary embolism
E Tuberculosis

19. Management of chest pain

A 61-year-old woman presents to the walk-in clinic with a history of tight, sternal chest pain "appearing out of the blue". Such episodes have occurred at different times throughout the day and rarely last longer than a few minutes. They do not correspond to hard exercise. The patient has no cardiac history to date. Her electrocardiogram (ECG) has not detected any abnormalities, and 2 days have passed since the last episode.

Which of the following is the next best step in her management?

A 24-hour ECG
B Admit to a ward
C Chest X-ray
D Echocardiogram
E Prescribe home oxygen

20. Barium enema

A 37-year-old woman is being investigated for weight loss and diarrhoea. Barium enema shows "cobble-stoning", rose thorn ulcers and colonic strictures at intermittent points throughout the colon. She is a smoker but has no other past medical history to date.

What is the most likely diagnosis?

A Coeliac disease
B Colonic carcinoma
C Crohn's disease
D Inflammatory bowel disease
E Ulcerative colitis

21. Cardiovascular examination

You are asked by your registrar to see a 40-year-old woman and report back your findings. On examination, you struggle to find an apex beat, although heart sounds 1 and 2 were audible with no murmur. On inspection, her electrocardiogram (ECG) is normal except for inverted P-waves in lead I.

What is the most likely reason for these findings?

A Dextrocardia
B Cardiomyopathy
C Mitral stenosis
D Myocardial ischaemia
E Pulmonary hypertension

22. Cauda equina syndrome

A 53-year-old man who has had some lower back pain and sciatica into his right leg for the past year presents with a 2-day history of leg weakness and severe pain.

On examination, which of the following signs does NOT make you think of cauda equina syndrome?

A Distended bladder
B Reduced anal tone
C Reduced reflexes in the ankles

D Saddle anaesthesia
E Upgoing plantars

23. Joint swelling

A 35-year-old man presents with a 3-week history of pain and swelling in the tips of his fingers. He has no history of bowel problems, recent infection or skin disease, but his brother has Crohn's disease. On examination you find several swollen, red, tender distal interphalangeal joints, and the nails have separated from the nailbed and have small pockmarks covering them. The rest of the examination is unremarkable.

Which of the following diagnoses is most likely?

A Enteropathic arthritis
B Osteoarthritis
C Psoriatic arthropathy

D Reactive arthritis
E Rheumatoid arthritis

24. Coeliac disease

Which of the following is a recognised complication of coeliac disease?

A Fistulae
B Intestinal lymphoma
C Primary sclerosing cholangitis

D Toxic megacolon
E Uveitis

25. Complications of alcoholic liver disease

You are called in the middle of the night to the surgical ward to see a 49-year-old man with known alcoholic liver disease admitted 2 days previously. He is shaking, sweating, tachycardic and apyrexial and believes he is seeing spiders crawling across the ceiling.

What is the most likely diagnosis?

A Alcohol intoxication
B Delirium tremens
C Bacterial peritonitis
D Fulminant hepatic necrosis
E Urinary tract infection

26. Diagnosis of abdominal pain

A 59-year-old woman with advanced metastatic breast cancer presents to the emergency department with severe abdominal pain. She has not opened her bowels for 7 days and feels constipated. She has also noticed that she has been passing water more frequently but has not been incontinent. On rectal examination there is no loss of anal tone and normal sensation.

What is the most likely diagnosis?

A Hypercalcaemia
B Hypocalcaemia
C Metastatic spread to the bowel
D Opiate-induced constipation
E Spinal cord compression

27. Disseminated intravascular coagulation

A 19-year-old female presents to the emergency department with a severe headache, photophobia, neck stiffness and a temperature. She is treated for bacterial meningitis with intravenous ceftriaxone. Blood cultures grow *Neisseria meningitides*. The next day, she starts bleeding from around her intravenous cannula and venepuncture sites.

Which of the following investigation results would you NOT expect in disseminated intravascular coagulation?

A Increased activated partial thromboplastin time (APTT)
B Increased fibrinogen
C Increased international normalised ratio (INR)
D Decreased haemoglobin
E Decreased platelets

28. Rectal bleeding

A 67-year-old man presents with painless rectal bleeding for the past 2 months. It occurs mainly on defecation and is bright red in the pan and on the toilet paper. A digital rectal examination is unremarkable.

What should your management be?

A Abdominal X-rays
B Review patient in 1 month to see if bleeding has stopped
C Routine bloods
D Routine outpatient appointment in 4–6 weeks
E Urgent 2-week outpatient referral

29. Diagnosis of cough

A 23-year-old final-year law student presents to the GP with a cough productive of foul green sputum. He also complains of breathlessness on exertion. He has had an average of five respiratory tract infections per year for the past 2 years. As a child, he could not tolerate dairy products. On examination, finger clubbing is present, and there is dullness to percussion of the right upper lung zone with widespread bilateral wheeze.

What is the most probable diagnosis?

A Asthma
B Coeliac disease
C Cystic fibrosis
D Immotile cilia syndrome
E Pneumonia

30. Diagnosis of gout

A 50-year-old overweight pub landlord presents with an acutely painful, swollen, red, hot first metatarsophalangeal joint on the left. You suspect gout.

Which of the following would confirm this on microscopy of a joint aspirate?

A Calcium pyrophosphate crystals
B Crystals of a rhomboid shape
C Crystals showing apple-green birefringence under polarised light
D Crystals showing negative birefringence under polarised light
E Crystals showing positive birefringence under polarised light

31. Investigation of shortness of breath

A 56-year-old man who has been recently diagnosed with sigmoid cancer and had a Hartmann's procedure is admitted to hospital with acute-onset shortness of breath. He denies any collapse or fainting. He has a past medical history of chronic obstructive pulmonary disease, hypertension, stroke and gout. His observations include temperature 37.2°C, pulse rate 106 bpm, blood pressure 110/74 mmHg, respiratory rate 25/min and saturations 87% on room air. There is no significant finding on chest examination. An electrocardiogram (ECG) shows sinus tachycardia with no ST elevation. A plain chest X-ray shows a small left pleural effusion.

Which of the following is the most appropriate diagnostic investigation?

A Magnetic resonance imaging (MRI) of the chest
B D-dimer level
C Computed tomographic pulmonary angiography
D Ventilation-perfusion scanning
E Echocardiography

32. Diagnosis of neurological dysfunction

A 27-year-old woman who works in the city as an investment banker presents with difficulty walking and a tremor in the right hand. It has come on over the last 4 days, and she is now unable to get to work safely. She denies any preceding respiratory or gastrointestinal infection or any abnormal stress at work or in her personal life; however, she says that 5 months ago she had some pain and blurring in the left eye for about 10 days, but she put that down to "sinusitis", kept working, and things returned to normal. Her grandfather, who died 2 years ago, had Parkinson's disease for some time, and she is concerned that this could be the same thing. On examination, in her arms, there is normal tone, power and sensation, but there is indeed a tremor in the right hand on testing coordination, which gets worse on approaching the target and is absent at rest. In the legs, there is normal power, but decreased light touch sensation bilaterally and a loss of vibration sense and proprioception up to the ankles.

What are you most concerned is the diagnosis?

A Acute disseminated encephalomyelitis
B Familial early-onset Parkinson's disease
C Guillain–Barré syndrome
D Multiple sclerosis
E Psychogenic neurological symptoms

33. Management of multiple sclerosis

A 33-year-old woman with multiple sclerosis (MS) is having problems with painful spasms and disabling spasticity in her left leg.

Which of the following medications is most likely to help?

A Baclofen
B Lactulose
C Modafinil
D Oxybutinin
E Propranolol

34. Diagnosis of stroke

A 65-year-old woman presents to hospital with sudden-onset left-sided weakness. She has type 2 diabetes, smokes 20 cigarettes a day and has high blood pressure. On examination, power in the left arm is 0 throughout, although the left leg shows a power of 3 at the hip and knee and 4 at the foot. Her reflexes are reduced throughout, and sensation is absent in the arm and reduced in the leg. In the cranial nerve examination, she is unable to see on her left side, and the lower half of her left face is weak (she can raise her eyebrow). There is no dysphasia.

Which vascular territory is affected?

A Left anterior cerebral artery
B Right anterior cerebral artery
C Right carotid artery
D Right middle cerebral artery
E Right posterior cerebral artery

35. Diagnosis of cough

A 45-year-old man presents to the GP with a 4-month history of a productive cough with exertional breathlessness. He denies haemoptysis or weight loss. He has a 20-pack/year smoking history. On examination, crackles are heard throughout the whole lung field.

What is most likely differential diagnosis?

A Asthma
B Chronic obstructive pulmonary disease
C Cystic fibrosis
D Idiopathic pulmonary fibrosis
E Lung cancer

36. Confusion

A 42-year-old woman presents to accident and emergency after being found wandering the streets by police. She is known to have bipolar disorder and takes lithium as a mood stabiliser. Which of the following does not increase the risk of lithium toxicity?

A Dehydration
B ACEi
C NSAIDs
D Renal disease
E Smoking

37. Diagnosis of chest pain

A 54-year-old woman presents to her GP complaining of repeated incidents of burning central chest pain. It mainly occurs when she lies down to go to bed at night. She is overweight with a body mass index of 40. She uses glyceryl trinitrate (GTN) occasionally, but it doesn't always relieve her symptoms. She doesn't report any shortness of breath or palpitations, and examination is unremarkable.

What is the most likely diagnosis?

A Angina
B Gastro-oesophageal reflux disease
C Myocardial infarction
D Pancreatitis
E Sleep apnoea

38. Eye assessment

A 44-year-old female has been diagnosed with neurosyphilis. What is the classic eye disorder associated with this condition?

A Argyll Robertson pupil
B Marcus Gunn pupil
C Kayser–Fleischer rings
D Anisocoria
E Brushfield spots

39. Electrocardiogram

A 78-year-old woman presents with palpitations that began an hour ago. She feels clammy to the touch. Whilst she is clutching your hand and telling you her past medical history, you check her observations on the bedside monitor. You notice that her heart rate is 230 bpm and regular. The QRS complexes are narrow, and no P-waves are noted.

What is the most likely arrhythmia?

A Atrial fibrillation
B Atrial flutter
C Atrioventricular node re-entry tachycardia
D Sinus tachycardia
E Ventricular tachycardia

40. Ingested foreign body

A 4-year-old boy swallowed a button battery while playing with his older siblings. He and his mother present to you, the GP, after a few hours. He is otherwise well in himself and has no previous medical history.

What should you do?

A Attempt gastric lavage
B Give laxatives to speed up the passage through the gut
C Manage expectantly and wait for it to pass naturally
D Refer immediately to hospital for evaluation and possible endoscopic retrieval
E Refer to social services

41. Management of acne

A 16-year-old boy presents with a 1-year history of acne affecting his face and upper back. He has tried over-the-counter creams and "a few creams prescribed by his GP", which turn out to be benzoyl peroxide and an antibiotic cream. None have worked, and the lesions have been getting worse. His friend had treatment with Roaccutane (isotretinoin), which sorted it out, and he is keen to try this. On examination he has acne on his face and upper back but without large pustules or scarring.

Which therapy might you recommend trying before isotretinoin?

A Oral cyproterone acetate
B Oral flucloxacillin
C Oral lymecycline
D Oral prednisolone
E Topical steroids

42. Statistics

A new blood test is being developed to help diagnose sarcoidosis. In a trial 100 patients have been tested. The trial produces 20 positive results and 80 negative results. Of the 20 positive results, 10 of them are false positives. Of the 80 negative results, 10 of them are false negatives.

What is the sensitivity of this test?

A 10%
B 25%
C 50%
D 75%
E 90%

43. Sexually transmitted infections

A 34-year-old woman who is known to be human immunodeficiency virus (HIV) positive presents with multiple lesions on her face. The lesions are raised and shiny, non-tender and around 3 mm in diameter. They have an umbilicated centre.

What is the most likely diagnosis?

A Herpes simplex
B Kaposi sarcoma
C Molluscum contagiosum
D Scabies
E Syphilis

44. Management of shortness of breath

A 49-year-old man presents to the emergency department with acute-onset right-sided pleuritic chest pain and shortness of breath. There was no associated trauma. He has a past medical history of chronic obstructive pulmonary disease, hypertension and diabetes mellitus. He smokes 40 cigarettes per day. His observations include temperature 37.2°C, pulse rate 95 bpm, blood pressure 150/92 mmHg, respiratory rate 24/min and saturations 92% on room air. A chest X-ray (CXR) shows a small rim of air (less than 2 cm) between the right lung edge and the chest wall.

Which of the following is the most appropriate first-line management?

A Admit to be observed only
B Intercostal tube drainage
C Medical pleurodesis
D Percutaneous needle aspiration
E Surgical pleurodesis

45. Signs of liver disease

A 52-year-old man with a history of alcohol excess presents to his GP because he cannot fully extend his ring finger on his right hand (neither actively nor passively). Since the finger is permanently partially flexed, he can no longer place his hand flat on a flat surface.

Which of the following is the most likely diagnosis?

A Asterixis
B Dupuytren contracture
C Palmar erythema
D Trigger finger
E Xanthelasma

46. Non-invasive ventilation

A 63-year-old man is admitted to the emergency department with severe dyspnoea. He is a long-standing smoker of 40 years. His observations are pulse rate 130 bpm, respiratory rate 36/min, oxygen saturation of 85% on 24% oxygen via a Venturi mask and temperature 38.2°C. Chest examination reveals reduced air entry on both lungs with coarse crackles on his left lower lobe. Despite immediate maximum standard medical treatment on controlled oxygen therapy, his arterial blood gas still shows persistent acidosis with a $PaCO_2$ of 8 kPa.

Which of the following would NOT be a required inclusion criterion for non-invasive ventilation?

A Ability to protect his airway
B Home oxygen use
C Patient's wishes considered
D Potential for recovery to quality of life acceptable to the patient
E Primary diagnosis of chronic pulmonary obstructive disease

47. Systemic lupus erythematosus

A 34-year-old woman with systemic lupus erythematosus (SLE) has had multiple miscarriages and now presents with a painful right swollen leg. A compression ultrasound scan confirms deep vein thrombosis.

Which blood test may now be indicated?

A Antiphospholipid antibodies
B Clotting factors
C Haemoglobin
D Pregnancy test
E Tumour markers

48. Medications in hyperkalaemia

A 74-year-old man with a history of hypertension, ischaemic heart disease and moderate congestive cardiac failure is admitted with a urinary tract infection and has developed acute renal failure. His potassium level is noted to be 5.5 mmol/L.

Which of his following medications may be contributing to the raised serum potassium level?

A Amlodipine
B Bendroflumethiazide
C Furosemide
D Simvastatin
E Spironolactone

49. Tumour markers

A 42-year-old woman attends to her GP complaining of non-specific abdominal pain and an increasing abdominal girth. She is found to have a large mass in her right lower abdomen and ascites on transvaginal ultrasound imaging.

Which of the following tumour markers would be most useful?

A CA 125
B Ca 15-3
C Ca 19-9
D CEA
E Beta-hCG

50. Parkinson's disease

Which of the following best describes the four cardinal signs of Parkinson's disease?

A Bradykinesia, mask-like facies, rigidity and tremor ~10–12 Hz
B Bradykinesia, micrographia, rigidity and tremor ~3–4 Hz
C Bradykinesia, postural hypotension, rigidity and tremor ~3–4 Hz
D Bradykinesia, postural instability, rigidity and tremor ~3–4 Hz
E Bradykinesia, postural instability, rigidity and tremor ~10–12 Hz

Practice paper 3: Answers

1. Acute coronary syndrome

C. 300 mg aspirin, 300 mg clopidogrel, oxygen (if hypoxic), heparin, beta-blocker, ACEi, with GTN spray morphine and metoclopramide PRN

Aspirin and clopidogrel should be initially given at 300 mg before reducing to 75 mg daily. Oxygen should be provided to all acutely unwell patients to facilitate oxygen delivery to tissues but should only be prescribed to hypoxic patients. Heparin will aid reperfusion to the heart, and fondaparinux is normally used in the setting of an non–ST-segment myocardial infarction (NSTEMI). Research has demonstrated both beta-blockers and angiotensin-converting enzyme inhibitors (ACEis) can be effective for secondary prevention and may be beneficial in reducing mortality rates.

2. Haematuria

B. Nephritic syndrome

Nephritic syndrome may be defined as a triad of haematuria (microscopic or macroscopic), hypertension and a reduction in the glomerular filtration rate. Along with the reduction in glomerular filtration rate and associated oliguria, oedema can be a feature, both peripheral and pulmonary, and pro-teinuria may also be present. This patient needs to be investigated for the cause of his nephritic syndrome and referred to a renal physician. As well as routine bloods, erythrocyte sedimentation rate (ESR) and C-reactive protein (CRP) need to be tested to look for an inflammatory cause. Serum and urine should be sent for electrophoresis to rule out myeloma and a renal screen, including complement (C3 and C4 – can be reduced in active lupus), antinuclear antibody, antineutrophil cytoplasm antibodies, anti-streptolysin-O titre (for post-streptococcal glomerulonephritis), anti–glomerular basement membrane antibodies (Goodpasture syndrome) and hepatitis serology. Urine should also be sent for 24-hour protein quantifica-tion (to look for concomitant nephrotic syndrome) and microscopy (to look for casts). The most common glomerulonephritis in the western world is IgA nephropathy (also known as Berger's disease). It usually affects young men following an upper respiratory tract infection. If there is ongoing renal impairment, immunosuppression is indicated.

DOI: 10.1201/9781003648222-6

Nephrotic syndrome is a triad of proteinuria, hypoalbuminemia and oedema – oedema is not a clinical feature here, and proteinuria was not found. Nephrotic syndrome, however, can often occur with nephritic syndrome – both are commonly caused by glomerulonephritides – and so it should be tested for with either a 24-hour urine protein quantification or a urine protein–creatinine ratio. Renal calculi can cause haematuria but is associated with severe pain.

Acute tubular necrosis is a form of acute renal injury usually following renal ischaemia due to dehydration, sepsis, hypotension or renal vascular disease. As such, it is common in hospital practice when pre-renal acute renal failure has not been sufficiently addressed. It can also be rarely caused by direct damage from drugs, including aminoglycosides and lithium. There is no reason to believe that any of these drugs or causes of renal hypoperfusion have taken place. Haematuria and hypertension are not typical features of acute tubular necrosis.

3. Heart failure

E. Digoxin is primarily a positive chronotropic drug

Digoxin, a cardiac glycoside extracted from the foxglove *Digitalis lanata*, which is an inotrope. By blocking the sodium/potassium pump, it causes a rise in intracellular sodium which, via sodium–calcium exchange, increases the intracellular concentration of calcium and hence contractility. As a result of the increased effort of myocardial contraction, atrioventricular node delay is increased, and heart rate is indirectly slowed.

Digoxin has been shown to relieve symptoms of heart failure without necessarily improving mortality, but it is the only inotrope that does not actually increase mortality. Digoxin has a narrow therapeutic index, and thus one must be vigilant for signs of toxicity such as headache, nausea, yellow-tinted vision and confusion. Toxicity may also cause life-threatening arrhythmia such as ventricular fibrillation. Toxicity is often triggered by electrolyte disturbance such as hypokalaemia, hypomagnesaemia or hypercalcaemia. One must ensure to look for precipitating factors and consider holding the next dose of digoxin or administering dedicated immunoglobulins.

Digitalis, from Latin *digitalis* = finger, with reference to the German name for foxglove, *Fingerhut* ("thimble")

4. Hodgkin's lymphoma

D. Stage IIIB

Hodgkin's lymphoma has a bimodal age distribution with peak incidences occurring in the third and sixth decades. It is usually of B-cell origin and is associated with a history of glandular fever. It classically presents with asymmetrical, painless lymphadenopathy, usually in the form of a single rubbery lymph node in the cervical, axillary or inguinal region that may become painful after alcohol ingestion. Disease spread to the mediastinal nodes may cause dyspnoea and superior vena cava obstruction. Approximately 20% of patients suffer systemic symptoms such as weight loss, sweating, fever, pruritus and general lethargy. These are known as "B" symptoms and are associated with a worse prognosis. Diagnosis is usually based on lymph node biopsy showing pathognomonic Reed–Sternberg cells (large malignant B cells). A CT scan often combined with a positron emission tomography (PET) scan is a key diagnostic tool used to assess spread and staging. The Ann Arbor system (I = one node region involved, II = ≥2 node regions on one side of diaphragm, III = incorporating both sides of diaphragm, IV = extra-nodal disease) is used for staging. The presence or absence of B symptoms is indicated in the staging by the suffix "A" (B symptoms absent) or "B" (B symptoms present). Early-stage disease is usually managed with radiotherapy alone. In advanced and bulky disease, the combination of radiotherapy and chemotherapy is often employed. The prognosis of Hodgkin's lymphoma is usually good, with a 70% chance of cure even in late-stage disease. Increasing age indicates a poorer prognosis.

Thomas Hodgkin, British physician (1798-1866)

Ann Arbor is a city in the US state of Michigan, where the Committee on Hodgkin Disease Staging classification met and revised the staging of lymphoma

5. Management of psoriasis

E. Ultraviolet therapy

Psoriasis is an autoimmune condition of patchy exaggerated skin growth. It typically involves the extensor regions of the body and presents with dry, scaly plaque. It has a high genetic predisposition with genes *PSORS1–9* mutated in roughly 50% of cases. One must emphasise to the patient that lifestyle changes, such as good sleep hygiene, reduce smoking/alcohol and balanced diet, can aid skin appearance. A range of topical therapies are available for psoriasis, and it can often take experimentation to find the right combination for each patient. Compliance with laborious application of creams is an issue, and patients differ widely in their approach. Tar is an effective therapy, especially crude tar, but stickiness, messiness and smell mean that most patients do not like using it. Dithranol is often used as a first-line medication in chronic plaque psoriasis; however, it can burn the skin (especially around the eyes) and can permanently stain clothes, so it needs to be used carefully. Potent steroids can be used, although they may induce a rebound phenomenon whereby lesions become worse than previously on stopping the topical steroids.

Phototherapy with exposure to specific ultraviolet (UV) light can be a useful next step in treatment for widespread psoriasis, as it can often rid a patient entirely of lesions without laborious cream application. There are two main types: UVB and psoralen-based UVA – both of which are given to reduce skin growth. The plaques often come back, however, at different rates and to different extents. It should not be given too many times in a person's life due to theoretical risk of skin cancers. It can result in sunburn, and so patients often start at a low dose and then increase the dose until the UV rays induce some erythema but not burn. Side effects and need for monitoring are markedly less than with the use of systemic therapies such as methotrexate, prednisolone and ciclosporin and biological agents such as infliximab, and these should be withheld for severe psoriasis refractory to topical and UV therapies.

6. Subarachnoid haemorrhage

B. Lumbar puncture (LP) immediately on admission is likely to show xanthochromia

Xanthochromia describes a straw-coloured appearance of the cerebrospinal fluid in subarachnoid haemorrhages caused by the presence of haemoglobin breakdown products and, as such, requires at least 6 hours before detection. LP at 12 hours is 95% sensitive when spectrophotometry is used to look for xanthochromia. Therefore, LP on admission may not be likely to show xanthochromia. Focal weakness may indeed ensue, either from haematoma or from arterial constriction or occlusion 4–12 days post-event – the surrounding blood clot, oedema and inflammatory factors induce vasoconstriction and further vessel inflammation, which could cause ischaemic brain damage. Of those making it into hospital, 10% present with new seizures. Extreme exertion and coitus may cause rupture of a cerebral aneurysm by sudden drastic increases in intracranial pressure. Unenhanced CT shows greater than 97% sensitivity in identifying subarachnoid haemorrhages within 6 hours of headache onset – blood enhances whiter than the surrounding brain matter due to the increased density of radio-opaque iron.

Xanthochromia, from Greek *xanthos* = yellow

7. Overdose and antidotes

E. Naloxone

This patient is suffering from a morphine overdose and is exhibiting the classic features of reduced responsiveness, pinpoint pupils and respiratory depression. This is a significant and potentially life-threatening overdose that will require treatment with naloxone. Naloxone competes with opiates for the mu receptors. It should be noted that naloxone has a very strong affinity for mu receptors and can therefore rapidly induce opiate withdrawal and trigger seizures. It is not uncommon for intravenous drug users to be extremely annoyed at medical staff for ruining their "high" with naloxone. Naloxone also has a shorter half-life compared to opiates, so repeated doses or an infusion may be required to maintain its beneficial effect.

Examples of antidotes and other medications used in overdose are provided in the following table.

- Antimuscarinic overdose   – Physostigmine
- Aspirin overdose   – Sodium bicarbonate
- Benzodiazepine overdose   – Flumazenil
- Beta-blocker overdose   – Atropine, glucagon
- Carbon monoxide poisoning   – Oxygen
- Digoxin overdose   – Digibind
- Heparin overdose   – Protamine sulphate
- Iron overdose   – Desferrioxamine
- Methanol overdose   – Ethanol
- Paracetamol overdose   – *N*-acetylcysteine
- Warfarin overdose   – Vitamin K

8. Pneumonia

E. Home with empirical antibiotic treatment when clinically stable

Community-acquired pneumonia can present as a wide spectrum of illness from mild and self-limiting to life-threatening. The CURB-65 score is used as an assessment of severity of pneumonia and helps decide the appropriate management. The recognition of mild disease with a low risk of complications enables patients to receive treatment at home, thus reducing inappropriate hospitalisation.

The CURB-65 score comprises five components, shown in the following table:

• Confusion	AMTS <8
• Urea	>7 mmol/L
• Respiratory rate	>30/min
• Blood pressure	Systolic <90 mmHg or diastolic 60 mmHg
• Age	>65 years

Each feature scores 1 point. Patients with a CURB-65 score of 0 or 1 point could receive home treatment with oral antibiotics. Patients with a CURB-65 score of 2 could be considered to receive short-stay hospital-supervised treatment. Patients with a CURB-65 score of ≥3 should be managed in the hospital as severe pneumonia (associated with a mortality rate of 22%), and if the CURB-65 score is 4 or 5, ICU admission should be considered. This gentleman's score is 1 and therefore E is the right answer.

9. Murmur

A. **Aortic stenosis**

Aortic stenosis can be a cause of shortness of breath and syncope due to reduced cardiac output. Back pain after a fall is common and is simply due to trauma in this case. Ejection systolic murmurs are the classic sign of aortic stenosis, as blood is ejected through the narrowed valvular orifice under high pressure, which generates turbulent noise. The most common cause of aortic stenosis is age-related calcification. Congenital bicuspid aortic valves are also vulnerable to calcification (prevalence 1–2%). Rheumatic fever (post-streptococcal autoimmune attack of valve tissue) also increases calcification. Treatment typically involves either surgical aortic valve replacement or transcatheter aortic valve implantation (TAVI). As TAVI may be done under local anaesthetic with sedation, it is suitable for those patients not fit for general anaesthetic. Many actors, including Arnold Schwarzenegger and Robin Williams, have had a valve replacement for aortic stenosis.

Aortic stenosis can also lead to heart failure, angina and Heyde's syndrome (colonic angiodysplasia and lower gastrointestinal bleeding associated with aortic stenosis). In the latter case, valve stenosis leads to von Willebrand disease (vWD) type 2A, possibly as the large von Willebrand platelet coagulation factor (vWF) molecule suffers shear stress as it traverses the aortic valve.

The types of vWD are as follows:

I   Heterozygous for gene defect, reduced levels of vWF
II   Normal vWF levels but structurally abnormal
IIA Abnormality in synthesis of vWF or with proteolysis
IIB Increased function of vWF, leading to spontaneous platelet binding
III   Homozygous for gene defect resulting in severe bleeding tendencies

Edward Heyde, contemporary American physician

Erik Adolf von Willebrand, Finnish paediatrician (1870-1949)

10. Skin lesions

B. **Pemphigoid**

Whilst we are not presented with a thorough history, and theoretically the man could have suffered multiple insect bites over the past few weeks, this would be extremely unusual, and even more so for the patient to not mention that he is living under constant assault. Stevens–Johnson syndrome (SJS) and toxic epidermal necrolysis (TEN) are both most often secondary to drug reactions, and we are not given a history of recent new medications started around the time of the start of disease. SJS is an extreme form of erythema multiforme (which presents with classic "target lesions"), with bullae and systemic involvement, including the pulmonary and renal systems, often with an extremely acute onset (rather than the subacute onset over weeks with which the man presented). In contrast to SJS (<10% body surface area affected), TEN involves rapid widespread loss (>30% body surface area) of large areas of the epidermis. Pemphigus does not present with such large tense blisters, but rather with flaccid blisters and erosions in erythematous patches. These burst easily and heal very slowly. The Nikolsky sign, in which the skin of the blister can be made to slide off with the push of a finger, is characteristic in pemphigus. Oral involvement is common. These are all in contrast to pemphigoid, which is far more common. They are both of autoimmune aetiology, and the pathological difference is the site of the splitting – in pemphigus, the split is within the epidermis, whereas in pemphigoid, the split is at the dermoepidermal junction. This is easily remembered as follows: pemphiguS = Superficial; pemphigoiD = Deep. Treatment of pemphigoid is with moderate doses of oral corticosteroids and often steroid-sparing immunosuppressants, such as azathioprine.

Pemphigus, from Greek *pemphix* = blister

Pyotr Nikolsky, Russian physician (1858–1940)

11. Antibiotics

A. Ceftriaxone and tendon rupture

Tendon rupture has been reported rarely with quinolones such as ciprofloxacin. The risk is increased in elderly patients and when corticosteroids are used concurrently. Co-amoxiclav can cause a derangement in liver function tests with a cholestatic picture, occasionally leading to jaundice, but withdrawal of the antibiotic usually leads to resolution. Macrolides such as erythromycin increase gastrointestinal motility and thus commonly cause diarrhoea; however, this has led to their intentional use as a prokinetic antiemetic. Gentamicin can cause significant renal damage, and hence the serum level of gentamicin is monitored during its use – increased levels suggest decreased urinary clearance due to nephrotoxicity, and the interval between doses should be increased. Nitrofurantoin is no longer commonly used, only being indicated for uncomplicated UTIs, and pulmonary hypersensitivity reactions leading to fibrosis can occur.

12. Scoring systems

E. Waterlow score

The Waterlow score is an important tool for assessing the risk of pressure sore development. Pressure sores are likely to develop in bedbound patients who have poor mobility, poor nutrition, incontinence and multiple co-morbidities. They can cause significant pain and, if they become infected, may lead to sepsis and even death. The Waterlow score is generally used by nurses during the admission of patients and is especially important in stroke victims, quadriplegics and comatose patients. Pressure sores require a multidisciplinary treatment approach and must involve tissue viability, physiologists, dieticians, general medical physicians (most likely geriatricians) and plastic surgeons.

Waterlow J. Pressure sores: a risk assessment card. *Nursing Times* 1985

13. Investigation of headache

D. Temporal artery biopsy

This woman has temporal arteritis. Giant cell arteritis (temporal arteritis) is an inflammatory vasculitis of the cranial branches arising from the aorta. It is most common in those over 50 and is twice as frequent in females. Clinical features include general malaise, temporal headache, scalp tenderness and jaw claudication. Eventually, visual disturbance or visual loss can occur due to ischaemic optic neuritis caused by arteritis of the ophthalmic artery (a branch of the internal carotid artery) and its branches of central retinal artery and posterior ciliary artery. On examination, an enlarged, tender, non-pulsatile temporal artery is seen on the affected side. Temporal artery biopsy is the definitive investigation (shows patchy granulomatous inflammation), but skip lesions may be present, and it is therefore possible that the histology is falsely negative. However, investigation should not delay treatment with steroids. A CT and MRI of the head would not tell us much about the state of the temporal arteries or whether they are inflamed. The erythrocyte sedimentation rate (ESR) is usually raised, but this is non-specific. Temporal artery ultrasound (TAUS), a non-invasive imaging technique, is being used as an adjunct to diagnosis.

14. Acutely swollen leg

A. Compartment syndrome

This woman has a tibial plateau fracture following a high-energy collision. Tibial plateau fractures are classified according to the Schatzker classification. Such injuries are a risk for compartment syndrome, and thus close regular neurovascular observations are essential. Compartment syndrome arises when the pressure in the fascial compartment of the leg (there are four compartments, each of which has its own neurovascular bundle) swells to the point where the pressure exceeds the capillary perfusion pressure. The eventual outcome if no intervention is made is an ischaemic, necrotic limb. This woman is displaying classic signs of compartment syndrome: a tight swollen limb with increasing pain worse on passive movement of the muscles within the compartment. Anything constricting should be removed from the limb with the leg elevated. A call should be made to the orthopaedic department immediately informing them of the surgical emergency. A group and save should be taken, the theatre booked and the patient consented and marked for fasciotomies.

15. Management of skin lesions

A. Chemotherapy

This man has a basal cell carcinoma (BCC). It is the most common skin cancer of which there are a variety of morphologies: nodular, superficial, morphoeic and pigmented. Risk factors include previous BCC, increasing age, family history, fair skin and genetic conditions such as Gorlin syndrome and xeroderma pigmentosa. The most common treatment is excision with 4-mm margins, as this not only removes all malignant cells but also enables the diagnosis to be made histologically. Excision is most often done under local anaesthetic, and complications are rare. In some circumstances, other treatment modalities can be used. Mohs micrographic surgery aims for extremely narrow excision margins, and histology is inspected at the time of excision to ensure the borders are clear, with repeat border trimmings until they are clear. This can be useful if there is limited local skin for closure or if there are nearby structures that are best avoided. Radiotherapy can be used to shrink lesions and reduce troublesome bleeding, often in cases where resection is difficult, either because of local invasion into certain structures or because the lesion is so large that flap reconstruction would be necessary and the patient is unsuitable for general anaesthetic. Topical 5-fluorouracil is commonly used for areas of skin with multiple or recurrent actinic keratoses and can be used in some instances of basal cell carcinoma, although this is a relatively recent development. Chemotherapy has severe side effects and with such a range of effective local treatment options, and as BCCs rarely metastasise, chemotherapy is entirely excessive and not indicated.

16. Fatigue

E. Obstructive sleep apnoea

Obstructive sleep apnoea is characterised by episodes of complete or partial upper airway obstruction during sleep. Patients experience episodic airway obstruction associated with oxyhaemoglobin desaturation and arousals from sleep. The symptoms of obstructive sleep apnoea include chronic snoring, insomnia, gasping and breath holding, non-refreshing sleep and daytime somnolence. The Epworth sleepiness scale score can aid diagnosis. Maxillomandibular anomalies, adenotonsillar hypertrophy, an increase in soft palatal and tongue tissue mass due to obesity and neuromuscular diseases with pharyngeal involvement leading to loss of dilator muscle tone are alternative causes of upper airway narrowing during sleep, which can lead to obstructive sleep apnoea. Treatment is usually by continuous positive airway pressure via a face mask during sleep.

17. Arterial blood gases

B. pH 7.22, pO$_2$ 18, pCO$_2$ 2.3, HCO$_3^-$ 10

One of the consequences of acute renal failure is metabolic acidosis, and given that this man's renal failure was precipitated by sepsis, this is likely to be more marked, as sepsis itself can cause metabolic acidosis. We are told that he was fluid resuscitated and treated with intravenous antibiotics; however, either the antibiotics have not been effective (and thus sepsis continues with vasodilation leading to renal hypoperfusion) or the fluid resuscitation has not been aggressive enough, or a combination of the two. His creatinine level has increased slightly, and his urine output is very low at 8 mL/hour. His breathing, which is described in the scenario – deep and laboured in the absence of any respiratory problem (clear chest, normal saturations on air) – is called "Kussmaul breathing" and is a natural response to acidosis and aims to reduce the amount of acidic carbon dioxide in the circulation. As can be seen, the only acidotic blood gas reading with a low pCO$_2$ ("partial respiratory compensation") is option B. Note that the bicarbonate level is low, indicating a metabolic nature to the acidosis. Option A appears to be a respiratory acidosis with no metabolic compensation. Option C appears to be a mixed respiratory and metabolic acidosis with a high pO$_2$ – this may be due to oxygen therapy. Option D shows carbon dioxide retention with full metabolic compensation – this may be the blood gas reading of a patient with chronic obstructive pulmonary disorder. Option E is respiratory alkalosis with no metabolic compensation – this picture may be caused by a panic attack with hyperventilation in the absence of any bodily disturbance.

18. Shortness of breath

B. Mesothelioma

Mesothelioma is a pleural tumour that is commonly associated with asbestos exposure. Shipyard workers, builders (mixing asbestos cement or fitting insulation), plumbers and electricians, who may be exposed to asbestos in their line of work, are more likely to develop asbestos-related lung disease. Breathlessness may be caused by a pleural effusion or circumferential pleural thickening. Computed tomography–guided biopsy or thoracoscopy provides a definitive diagnosis. The prognosis of malignant mesothelioma is poor. The median survival in a variety of studies is between 8 and 14 months from diagnosis.

For more information, see the British Thoracic Society statement on malignant mesothelioma in the UK. *Thorax* 2007; 62(Suppl2): ii1-19.

19. Management of chest pain

A. 24-hour ECG

This chest pain is probably cardiac in origin, secondary to paroxysmal tachycardia. This is best detected by 24-hour ECG. It lacks the correlation with effort of new-onset, stable angina secondary to coronary vascular disease. Any instance of tight chest pain or chest pain of sternal origin should be taken very seriously indeed. It is only because in this case she has not experienced the pain for at least 48 hours that a troponin blood test is not indicated – after this time it will not distinguish between a myocardial infarction (MI) and angina. An echocardiogram will detect structural cardiac lesions, especially at the valvular level, but will not identify arrhythmias. Home oxygen is usually prescribed for patients with respiratory disease and chronic hypoxia after a full assessment; a cardiac patient so hypoxic that they need supplemental oxygen should not be sent home. Analysis of the 24-hour or ambulatory ECG will indicate the source of the tachycardia, i.e. supraventricular or ventricular (much more serious), which will in turn indicate a management plan that may include permanent pacing.

20. Barium enema

C. Crohn's disease

Barium enemas have largely been superseded by more advanced imaging and better endoscopy techniques but often still appear in exam questions. Described earlier are the signs of Crohn's disease. Crohn's disease is a relapsing inflammatory bowel disease affecting the whole of the gastrointestinal (GI) tract of which the characteristic feature is transmural granuloma. It typically presents with weight loss, anaemia and diarrhoea, although extra-intestinal features such as iritis, clubbing and erythema nodosum are seen. Such patients are at risk of peri-anal disease. Investigations with blood tests, faecal calprotectin, contrast studies and endoscopic biopsies should be undertaken. The main differential is ulcerative colitis, which would produce continuous changes from the rectum proximally and show a loss of haustra on plain film and a colon appearing shortened. Smoking is also a protective factor for ulcerative colitis. The classic representation of colonic carcinoma is the stricturing "apple-core lesion". Coeliac disease is a condition involving the small bowel and so should not show signs on barium enema.

21. Cardiovascular examination

A. Dextrocardia

Inverted P-waves can be caused by dextrocardia or by the natural cardiac pacemaker being situated elsewhere in the atrium other than the sinoatrial node. In dextrocardia, the apex beat would be palpable on the right. Typical ECG features include right axis deviation, positive QRS in aVR with global negativity in lead I (inverted P-wave, negative QRS and inverted T-wave) and absent R-wave progression in the chest leads.

Dextrocardia is a congenital condition, meaning a normal heart is situated unusually rightward (dextrocardia of embryonic arrest and, as the name grimly suggests, is associated with malformations), or, less commonly, occurring as a mirror image on the right (dextrocardia situs inversus). If all internal organs are mirrored, it is known as dextrocardia situs inversus totalis (this is very rare). The latter two conditions are benign, although they can occur in conjunction with primary ciliary dyskinesia (Kartagener syndrome).

Dextrocardia, from Latin *dextro* = right + Greek *cardia* = heart

Manes Kartagener, Polish physician (1897-1957)

22. Cauda equina syndrome

E. Upgoing plantars

The spinal cord ends with the conus medullaris around L2, below which the dural sac simply contains the cauda equina, nerve roots that will exit at the lower lumbar and sacral spine. Saddle anaesthesia is due to compression of the sensory fibres leaving the spine at S3–S5. The bladder may be distended, as detrusor motor paralysis and sensory loss lead to urinary retention. The lower motor neurone nature of the weakness reduces the anal tone and may lead to reduced or absent ankle reflexes. Cauda equina syndrome is an emergency and must be discussed urgently with neurosurgery. It is typically caused by disc prolapse, malignancy, trauma, abscess or haematoma and requires urgent whole-spine MRI prior to discussion with the on-call neurosurgical team.

Cauda equina, from Latin *cauda* = tail + *equus* = horse

23. Joint swelling

C. Psoriatic arthropathy

In enteropathic arthritis, flares happen at the same time as flares of inflammatory bowel disease, and so given the absence of any such symptoms, this diagnosis can be excluded. It also most commonly affects large joints of the lower limbs. Diffuse osteoarthritis affecting distal interphalangeal joints occurs far more frequently in postmenopausal females, and 35 years of age is very young for osteoarthritis. Psoriatic arthropathy has a typical onset between the ages of 25 and 40 years, and in 20% of patients it predates the appearance of psoriatic skin lesions (and in 5% there is never any skin involvement).

It is a diffuse disease category and there are five major patterns:

1. Distal interphalangeal joint predominance (seen here, most common in men and most strongly associated with nail changes – onycholysis is the separation of the nail from the bed seen here, and pitting is also seen)
2. Asymmetrical oligoarthritis (commonly featuring dactylitis or "sausage fingers")
3. Symmetrical polyarthritis (resembling rheumatoid arthritis but less severe and not associated with nodules or other manifestations; it is more common in females)
4. Psoriatic spondylitis (less severe than ankylosing spondylitis)
5. Arthritis mutilans (also seen with rheumatoid arthritis; erosion of bone and cartilage in the fingers leads to telescoping)

Psoriatic arthropathy is typically managed in a stepwise manner with non-steroidal anti-inflammatory drugs (NSAIDs), disease-modifying anti-rheumatic drugs (DMARDs) and biological agents. Reactive arthritis is commonly found following dysentery or *Chlamydia* infection and has a marked preponderance for lower limb involvement. It is associated with conjunctivitis in 50% of cases and a non-specific urethritis (hence the mnemonic "Can't see, can't pee, can't bend a knee"). It is far more common in men than in women (15:1). Enteropathic arthritis, psoriatic arthropathy, reactive arthritis and ankylosing spondylitis are the seronegative spondyloarthropathies and are heavily associated with *HLA-B27*, an immune histocompatibility gene (hence the relevance of the brother with Crohn's disease).

24. Coeliac disease

B. Intestinal lymphoma

There is an 80-fold increased relative risk of intestinal lymphoma in coeliac disease compared to the normal population. These are predominantly T-cell–derived lymphomas, and the risk is reduced with effective gluten exclusion. The other complications and associations listed are relevant to the inflammatory bowel diseases.

25. Complications of alcoholic liver disease

B. Delirium tremens

Delirium tremens is a syndrome of delirium, autonomic activation and agitation brought on by acute detoxification from alcohol. It is a terrifying and potentially life-threatening confusional state, with a 35% mortality rate if left untreated. It can progress to seizures and heart arrhythmias. In these patients it is important to monitor their vital signs, as they can have precipitous drops in their blood pressure. Treatment is with benzodiazepines, such as chlordiazepoxide. Intravenous Pabrinex (a high-potency vitamin solution) and oral thiamine should be initiated in addition to chlordiaz-epoxide. He should be managed, if possible, as any patient with delirium: quiet side room with visual prompts of time orientation. One must be aware of delirium tremens when considering consent for any future surgical procedure.

26. Diagnosis of abdominal pain

A. Hypercalcaemia

Hypercalcaemia should always be suspected in patients with vague abdominal symptoms and known metastatic carcinoma, especially in malignancies prone to spread to the bone (breast, bronchus, kidney, prostate, thyroid and myeloma). Obviously in this scenario the most important differential to exclude is spinal cord compression. As well as malignancy, hypercalcaemia may be caused by primary hyperparathyroidism. Hypercalcaemia is said to cause "bones, abdominal groans, psychiatric moans and stones"; this refers to changes in bone metabolism, abdominal pain, psychiatric symptoms and increased frequency of calcium stones. Treatment is initially supportive with good rehydration and identification and treatment of the underlying cause where possible. Bisphosphonates can also be used to lower serum calcium.

27. Disseminated intravascular coagulation

B. Increased fibrinogen

Meningococcal septicaemia can cause disseminated intravascular coagulation, as can a number of other infections (including *Escherichia coli*, *Streptococcus pneumoniae* and malaria) and other conditions, including lung and pancreatic cancer. Diffuse endothelial damage leads to widespread tissue factor expression, thus activating intravascular coagulation and consuming platelets, factors V and VIII and fibrinogen. Therefore, the patient enters a haemorrhagic state. The INR and APTT both increase, as both depend on factor V and fibrinogen. Platelets are used up in the coagulation and thus fall, and haemoglobin is likely to fall with ongoing blood loss. However, the fibrinogen levels on the bloods should decrease, as it is used in the intravascular coagulation. Treatment of the cause should be combined with platelets and/or fresh frozen plasma as indicated by blood results and the clinical scenario.

28. Rectal bleeding

E. Urgent 2-week outpatient referral

In the scenario this bleeding may well be secondary to haemorrhoids, in that it is painless bleeding at the end of defecation. However, above the age of 60, any rectal bleeding warrants urgent investigation to rule out rectal carcinoma. Other criteria for urgent referral include a change of bowel habits for 6 weeks or more, unexplained iron-deficiency anaemia and any palpable mass. Bowel cancer is the fourth most common cancer in the UK.

29. Diagnosis of cough

C. Cystic fibrosis

Cystic fibrosis (CF) is the most common autosomal recessive condition in the Caucasian populations in the UK, affecting one in 2500 live births. CF is caused by an abnormal gene coding for the cystic fibrosis transmembrane regulator protein (CFTR), located on chromosome 7. CFTR is a cAMP-dependent chloride channel. In CF this is defective and leads to the defective transport of chloride and water across epithelial cells. The most common mutation in CF is the ΔF508 mutation. The poor transport of chloride ions and water across epithelial cells of the respiratory and pancreatic exocrine glands in CF results in an increased viscosity of secretions. The range of presentations is varied, including recurrent chest infections, failure to thrive due to malabsorption and liver disease. In the neonatal period, infants may present with prolonged neonatal jaundice, bowel obstruction (meconium ileus) or rectal prolapse.

The gold standard investigation for CF is the sweat test. The abnormal function of sweat glands results in the excess concentration of sodium chloride (NaCl) in sweat. Sweat is stimulated by pilocarpine iontophoresis, collected on filter paper and analysed.

Normal sweat NaCl concentration: 10–14 mmol/L

Sweat NaCl concentration in CF: 80–125 mmol/L

A result of $\geq$60 mmol/L is diagnostic in most cases, especially in infants. At least two sweat tests should be performed, as diagnostic errors and false positives are common.

Management options in CF include physiotherapy (for respiratory secretions), antibiotics (for prophylaxis and treatment of lung infections) and pancreatic enzyme supplements (to prevent malabsorption). Complications include diabetes mellitus, hepatic cirrhosis, infertility in males, severe pulmonary hypertension and cor pulmonale and chronic lung infections (*Pseudomonas aeruginosa* and *Burkholderia cepacia*). Many cases of CF are now being picked up early since the introduction of a national screening programme assessing immunoreactive trypsin (IRT) levels on the Guthrie card at day 8 of life. IRT is a pancreatic enzyme whose levels are raised in CF.

30. Diagnosis of gout

D. Crystals showing negative birefringence under polarised light

Calcium pyrophosphate crystals cause pseudogout. These are positively birefringent crystals and rhomboidal ("brick-shaped"). Apple-green birefringence under polarised light is seen in tissues with amyloid deposits and stained with Congo red. The negatively birefringent crystals of gout are spindle or needle shaped.

Gout occurs secondary to the deposition of uric acid crystals in the joint. It is most common in older, obese male drinkers with hypertension, ischaemic heart disease and diabetes. Other risk factors include cytotoxic drugs, diuretic use and Lesch–Nyhan syndrome (gout + mental retardation + self-mutilating behaviour). Acute episodes of gout can be precipitated by trauma, illness, stress and thiazide diuretics. Acute gout usually presents with sudden pain, swelling and redness in the first metatarsophalangeal joint, although 25% of cases occur in the knee. Diagnosis is by joint aspiration, which shows negatively birefringent needle-shaped crystals. Acute gout is treated with non-steroidal anti-inflammatory drugs (NSAIDs, e.g. indomethacin, diclofenac) or colchicine. Side effects of colchicine, including diarrhoea, limit its use; however, it is useful in patients unable to take NSAIDs such as those with asthma, heart failure or peptic ulcers. If both NSAIDs and colchicine are not tolerated, one may reconsider the diagnosis or, if definitely gout, consider canakinumab (interleukin-1 beta inhibitor). As well as lifestyle advice, prophylaxis is with allopurinol, a xanthine oxidase inhibitor that slows the production of uric acid. This is offered to patients who have recurrent gout or chronic gout, who are using cytotoxic therapy and those with Lesch–Nyhan syndrome. Allopurinol should not be prescribed within 1 month of an attack of gout, as it may precipitate a further attack. In patients allergic to allopurinol, probenecid is used as prophylaxis.

Other forms of gout are chronic tophaceous gout (the accumulation of urate in cartilage, often the ear and Achilles tendon) and gout nephropathy (urate deposition in the kidneys resulting in acute renal failure and the formation of urate stones).

Gout, from Latin *gutta* = a drop

The ancient physician Galen thought that gout was caused by a small drop of the four humours in unbalanced proportions leaking into the joint space. The four humours - black bile, yellow bile, phlegm and blood - were thought to be the four basic substances of the human body, disturbances of which resulted in disease.

31. Investigation of shortness of breath

C. Computed tomographic pulmonary angiography

Most pulmonary embolisms (PEs; 75%) derive from a deep vein thrombosis; however, they may also occur following amniotic or fat emboli. Features include acute-onset pleuritic chest pain and shortness of breath, often with fever and tachycardia. The chest X-ray may show a wedge-shaped opacity due to consolidation associated with pulmonary infarction (Hampton hump), or it may show no abnormalities. The Westermark sign is a focus of oligaemia on X-ray distal to an occluded blood vessel. The ECG most commonly demonstrates a sinus tachycardia, although the S1Q3T3 pattern is characteristic (S-wave in lead I, Q-wave and inverted T-wave in lead III). An arterial blood gas reading reveals type 1 respiratory failure (normal pH, low pO_2). D-dimers are a breakdown product of clots: a low D-dimer can be used to exclude a PE, but a high level does not confirm it. A spiral CT (computed tomography pulmonary angiography [CTPA]) is the best investigation; however, a ventilation/perfusion scan (V/Q scan) may be used if the patient has a contrast allergy or should not be exposed to radiation. Patients with a confirmed PE are started on heparin or low-molecular-weight heparin and then either offered warfarin or rivaroxaban for 3–6 months. If patients are unsuitable for oral anticoagulation, an inferior vena cava (IVC) filter may be used. Patients who have suffered a massive PE may need urgent thrombolysis. Echocardiography is useful in diagnosis of massive PE. Acute dilatation of the right heart is usually present in massive PE with visible thrombus seen.

32. Diagnosis of neurological dysfunction

D. Multiple sclerosis

Whilst she is concerned that this is Parkinson's disease, and there are some rare cases of early-onset familial Parkinson's disease caused by mutations in a single gene (for instance, alpha-synuclein, the misfolded protein that makes up Lewy bodies), not only is 27 still extremely young, but the clinical picture does not sound like Parkinson's disease. There is no sensory loss in Parkinson's disease, and the tremor is absent at rest and gets worse on movement (the opposite of the parkinsonian tremor). The tremor in fact sounds like an intention tremor. Regarding the symptoms being possibly psychogenic, this is common in young patients (especially female); however, there is no history of psychological abnormality, and the examination findings seem reliably reproducible and are consistent with certain anatomical lesions. Psychogenic neurology is often a diagnosis of exclusion.

The lack of an identified preceding infection does not preclude a postinfectious condition, either peripheral (Guillain–Barré) or central (acute disseminated encephalomyelitis [ADEM]), and indeed the subacute onset could fit with such a diagnosis. However, the intention tremor in the arm with lack of sensory symptoms or examination findings is most likely cerebellar in nature, and the cerebellum is not commonly affected in Guillain–Barré syndrome.

Multiple sclerosis (MS) is the most common organic central nervous system disorder in the young and affects women more than men, so this is the most likely diagnosis. MS is an autoimmune condition which attacks the myelin sheath of nerves, with lesions disseminated in time and place. Over time, scarring of the nerves leads to slowing of conduction of nerve impulses. The feature in the history that supports this is the episode of visual blurring and eye pain (optic neuritis). In the optic nerve, the axons conducting messages from the cone cells (colour vision and high-acuity central vision) are myelinated, but those conducting messages from rod cells (dark vision and peripheral vision) are not, and so central vision and colour vision are more commonly affected. The eye pain is commonly exacerbated on eye movement as the inflamed optic nerve sheath is stretched; however, this episode was mild, and the hard-working patient has worked through it and forgotten such detail, so this is uncertain.

MS causes systemic symptoms, and in addition to optic neuritis patients may complain of tremor, loss of sensation and proprioception in the lower limbs, incontinence and impotence. Management is typically with steroids and disease-modifying agents such as interferon beta and glatiramer. MS is a life-changing condition, and patients should be monitored in the community. The mainstay of management includes management of chronic pain, depression, muscle spasms, incontinence and pressure sores.

33. Management of multiple sclerosis

A. Baclofen

Baclofen is a gamma-amino-butyric acid (GABA)–derived drug commonly used as an antispasmodic. Oxybutinin is an anticholinergic used in detrusor instability and urinary continence issues in multiple sclerosis (MS). MS sufferers can become constipated, so lactulose (an osmotic laxative) can help. Modafinil is a stimulant drug sometimes used in MS to combat fatigue. Beta-blockers such as propranolol can help with tremor.

34. Diagnosis of stroke

D. Right middle cerebral artery

The cranial nerve examination shows an upper motor neurone pattern of weakness on the same side as the limb weakness and a homonymous hemianopia on the same side, which localises this stroke to the cerebral hemisphere rather than the brainstem. For that reason, the posterior cerebral artery cannot be the affected artery. The left side of the body is affected, so it must be the right cerebral hemisphere – ruling out any artery on the left. That leaves us the right carotid, anterior cerebral or middle cerebral arteries. The arm and face being affected rules out the anterior cerebral artery, and the relative sparing of the leg (especially distal) indicates that it is the right middle cerebral artery territory that is affected. The right middle cerebral artery passes anterolaterally from the circle of Willis to lie on the outside of the hemisphere before turning to run posteriorly in the Sylvian fissure, supplying the lateral part of all four lobes.

35. Diagnosis of cough

B. Chronic obstructive pulmonary disease

This man has chronic obstructive pulmonary disease (COPD), as evidenced by a decreasing exercise tolerance and productive cough on a background of a smoking history. COPD is a chronic progressive disorder characterised by airflow obstruction. The obstruction may be partially (but not completely) reversible with bronchodilators. COPD encompasses bronchitis and emphysema. Chronic bronchitis is defined as cough with sputum for most days of a 3-month period for 2 consecutive years. Emphysema is a pathological diagnosis of permanent destructive enlargement of the alveoli.

Smoking is the main risk factor, and 15% of smokers develop COPD. The pathology includes hypertrophy of the goblet cells and decreased cilia with loss of alveoli elastic recoil. The persistent hypoxaemia seen in COPD results in pulmonary vascular hypertension, which leads to cor pulmonale. Features of COPD include a productive cough (worse in the mornings), recurrent respiratory tract infections, exertional dyspnoea, expiratory wheeze and bibasal crepitations. Examination may also reveal tracheal tug, intercostal in-drawing, a barrel chest (increased anterior–posterior diameter), pursed lips, central cyanosis, carbon dioxide retention (flapping tremor, bounding pulse and warm peripheries) and right heart failure.

COPD is diagnosed by demonstrating a forced expiratory volume in 1 second (FEV_1) of <80% and an FEV_1/VC (vital capacity) ratio of <70% with little variation in peak flow. The lung capacity and residual volume are increased. Arterial blood gases typically show hypoxia and hypercapnia. A chest X-ray shows hypertranslucent lung fields, a flat diaphragm, bullae and prominent hila. Management options include stopping smoking, antibiotics for infections, regular anticholinergics (ipratropium) and a salbutamol inhaler as required. Smoking cessation can be helped by bupropion, which is prescribed 2 weeks before stopping. Long-term oxygen therapy (LTOT) of 1–4 L/min via nasal cannulae is given for patients with severe COPD who have given up smoking and who have a pO_2 < 7.3 kPa and FEV_1 < 1.5 L. Acute exacerbations of COPD are diagnosed when patients complain of worsening exercise tolerance, increasing sputum volume and increasing sputum purulence. Acute exacerbations of COPD are treated with controlled oxygen therapy, nebulised salbutamol and ipratropium bromide, oral prednisolone and prophylactic low-molecular-weight heparin. If CO_2 is rising or the patient is acidotic despite adequate oxygen therapy, consider ventilator support.

36. Confusion

E. Smoking

Lithium is commonly used for the management of bipolar disorder. It is an effective medication, although it has a narrow therapeutic index (0.6–1). Lithium clearance is predominately via renal excretion, and thus a variety of factors may increase the serum levels and risk toxicity. Angiotensin-converting enzyme inhibitors (ACEis), non-steroidal anti-inflammatory drugs (NSAIDs), diuretics, dehydration and known renal disease contribute to an increased risk of toxicity. It typically presents with tremor, diarrhoea, vomiting and confusion and may lead to cardiac arrhythmias and cerebellar dysfunction. Treatment involves withholding lithium, hydration and gastric decontamination.

37. Diagnosis of chest pain

B. Gastro-oesophageal reflux disease

Differentiating gastro-oesophageal reflux disease (GORD) from a cardiac cause of pain can be extremely difficult. In this case the salient features are that the pain occurs on lying down to go to sleep. Although in unstable angina this may occur, you would also expect a patient to report pain on increased exertion as well. A glyceryl trinitrite (GTN) spray may relieve both GORD and angina, as the nitrates cause smooth muscle relaxation in the oesophagus as well as coronary arteries.

GORD is associated with obesity, smoking, alcohol, hernias and pregnancy. Patients generally present with intermittent pain, or heartburn, which may be related to lifestyle factors such as large meals or alcohol. Medications can also contribute and should be reviewed. Endoscopy is not usually indicated for the diagnosis in young, otherwise healthy patients; however, urgent referrals should be considered in anyone over the age of 55 with new-onset symptoms or warning signs of weight loss, gastrointestinal (GI) bleeding or anaemia. Management of dyspepsia is modification of lifestyle factors, including weight loss, and pharmacological treatment with proton pump inhibitors. One should be tested for *Helicobacter pylori* and treated accordingly. Complications of long-standing reflux are the development of Barrett's oesophagus, formation of strictures and oesophageal cancer.

38. Eye assessment

A. Argyll Robertson pupil

Syphilis is a sexually transmitted infection (STI) caused by *Treponema pallidum*. Recent public health data has shown a 14% increase in annual incidence. It has a wide spectrum of disease, ranging from a painless genital ulcer known as a chancre, widespread macular-papular rash and neuro-logical sequelae. The classic eye pathology is known as an Argyll Robertson pupil, which accommodates to nearby structures but does not react to light. A Marcus Gunn pupil is caused by an optic nerve lesion, which presents as a relative afferent pupillary defect. Anisocoria is a difference in the size of pupils and, although physiological, may also be caused by Horner's syn-drome. Kayser–Fleischer rings are seen in Wilson's disease and are a sign of excess copper deposition within the cornea. Brushfield spots are classic of Down syndrome and present with white spots on the iris.

39. Electrocardiogram

C. Atrioventricular node re-entry tachycardia

Arrhythmias can be categorised as sinus node abnormalities, supraven-tricular or ventricular arrhythmias. Sinus bradycardia and sinus tachy-cardia are common sinus node abnormalities, and the P-waves remain associated with QRS complexes, confirming normal functioning of cardiac conduction. The causes usually lie outside of the heart. Supraventricular arrhythmias include atrial ectopic beats, paroxysmal tachycardias (narrow complexes generated below the sinoatrial node but above the ventricles), Wolff–Parkinson–White syndrome (a separate pathway to the atrioven-tricular node [AVN] allows pre-excitation and re-entry), atrial flutter and atrial fibrillation. Atrial flutter is caused by a re-entry pathway allowing rapid refiring of the ventricles: a rate of 300/min is typical. The AVN will often block some of the beats, and additional P-waves appear at a regular rate of 300/min between QRS complexes. Atrial fibrillation is characterised by an irregular heart rate. Ventricular arrhythmias include ventricular ectopic beats, torsade de pointes, ventricular tachycardia and ventricular fibrillation. A broad QRS complex tachycardia indicates a ventricular arrhythmia (or a supraventricular arrhythmia with bundle branch block). AVN re-entry tachycardia occurs when two pathways co-exist within the AVN. The two pathways may have differing delays, which, in total, present a raised heart rate of between 140 and 220 bpm. These paroxysms can be managed with adenosine or verapamil to cause an iatrogenic AVN delay.

40. Ingested foreign body

D. Refer immediately to hospital for evaluation and possible endoscopic retrieval

Swallowing of foreign objects is a relatively common presentation in chil-dren. Most non-harmful objects can be managed expectantly and should pass through the gastrointestinal tract within 5–7 days. The parents should be asked to look for the object to ensure it passes. Anything that is poten-tially toxic, such as batteries and sharp objects, or anything especially large, should be immediately referred to hospital for potential removal under endoscopy. The narrowest part of the gastrointestinal (GI) tract is the oesophagus, and this is the most common site of impaction. If a battery becomes lodged in the oesophagus, removal is advised to avoid the small chance of oesophageal perforation. Once the object has passed into the stomach, the chances of impaction are low.

41. Management of acne

C. Oral lymecycline

Cyproterone acetate is an anti-androgen that may only be given to women, so it is contraindicated here. Topical steroid creams may be used when there are focal severe lesions, whereas this patient has diffuse but non-severe lesions. Oral prednisolone may only be used in severe cases, often where isotretinoin has not been fully effective. Systemic antibiotic therapy can be effective at clearing up acne and often should be prescribed for over 6 months. Fat-soluble antibiotics are better delivered to the target (therefore, penicillins are not preferred). Rather, tetracyclines or sometimes erythromycin is used.

42. Statistics

C. 50%

The sensitivity of an investigation is its ability to detect a truly positive result. It is calculated as follows:

$$\text{Sensitivity} = \text{number of true positives}/(\text{number of true positives} + \text{number of false negatives}) \times 100$$

$$\text{In this case} = 10/(10 + 10) \times 100 = 50\%$$

43. Sexually transmitted infections

C. Molluscum contagiosum

Molluscum contagiosum is caused by DNA-containing poxvirus. Spread is by sexual contact, personal contact and fomites (an inanimate object that is contaminated with disease-causing microorganisms, such as a used towel). Hemispherical papules of 2–5 mm diameter that are pearly, raised and firm develop on the face, abdomen, buttocks and genitals. There is a latent period of 15–50 days. Spontaneous regression generally occurs, but lesions can be present for several months, and topical salicylic acid or imiquimod cream may shorten the duration. Lesions can be extensive and persistent in immunocompromised patients, including those with HIV.

Molluscum, from Latin *molluscus* = a fungus (a particular type that grows on maple trees)

44. Management of shortness of breath

B. Intercostal tube drainage

Pneumothorax is the presence of air in the pleural space. It can occur spontaneously in healthy people (primary spontaneous pneumothorax) or in patients with pre-existing lung disease (secondary spontaneous pneumothorax). It can also result from iatrogenic injury or trauma to the lung or chest wall. Management of pneumothorax depends on the size of pneumothorax, clinical symptoms and underlying lung disease. The size of pneumothorax is divided into small or large depending on the size of the visible rim of air between the lung margin and the chest wall: <2 cm or ≥2 cm. Observation without any intervention is advised for small, closed and mildly symptomatic primary spontaneous pneumothoraces, and these patients do not require hospital admission. In patients with asymptomatic small secondary pneumothoraces, it is recommended to be admitted into hospital for observation. In patients with symptomatic primary or secondary pneumothoraces, active intervention is required, as it may herald tension pneumothorax. Simple aspiration is recommended as first-line treatment for all primary pneumothoraces requiring intervention and mildly symptomatic small (<2 cm) secondary pneumothoraces. Intercostal tube drainage is recommended as first-line intervention in other symptomatic secondary pneumothoraces, as they may cause respiratory failure. Tube drainage is also used if simple aspiration fails to control symptoms in any pneumothorax. Pleurodesis is to be considered to prevent recurrence in primary or secondary spontaneous pneumothorax.

45. Signs of liver disease

B. Dupuytren contracture

The palmar aponeurosis extends from the palmaris longus to each digit. It protects the underlying muscles and neurovascular structures within the hand. Dupuytren contracture is a progressive fibroplasia of the palmar aponeurosis that results in a flexion contracture of the fingers – most commonly the ring and little fingers. It is characterised by the myofibroblast, and risk factors include male sex, age, a positive family history, diabetes mellitus, alcoholic cirrhosis, phenytoin use, trauma, acquired immunodeficiency syndrome (AIDS), Peyronie's disease (idiopathic fibrosis of the corpus cavernosum) and Ledderhose disease (fibrosis of the plantar fascia, resulting in a similar deformity). On examination the thickened palmar aponeurosis can be felt and will lead to a positive tabletop test (the hand cannot lie flat). Many treatment options exist and include collagenase injections, needle aponeurotomy and surgical excision of the thickened part of the aponeurosis. One must be made aware of the high recurrence rate when consenting to surgical release.

Guillaume Dupuytren, French surgeon (1777-1835)

46. Non-invasive ventilation

B. Home oxygen use

Non-invasive ventilation is now widely used in patients with chronic hypercapnic respiratory failure caused by chest wall deformity, neuro-muscular disease or impaired central respiratory drive. It has a number of potential advantages, particularly the avoidance of tracheal intubation with its associated mortality and morbidity from problems such as pneu-monia. According to the guidelines on non-invasive ventilation in chronic obstructive pulmonary disease (management of acute type 2 respiratory failure published by the British Thoracic Society), the inclusion criteria are: (1) primary diagnosis of chronic obstructive pulmonary disease (COPD) exacerbation (known diagnosis or history and examination consistent with diagnosis); (2) ability to protect airway; (3) patient is conscious and cooperative; (4) potential for recovery to quality of life acceptable to the patient; and (5) patient's wishes are considered. There is evidence to sup-port the use of non-invasive ventilation in patients who are comatose sec-ondary to COPD-induced hypercapnia in which endotracheal intubation is deemed inappropriate.

47. Systemic lupus erythematosus

A. Antiphospholipid antibodies

Antiphospholipid antibodies (anticardiolipin or lupus anticoagulant) are present in 30% of systemic lupus erythematosus (SLE) sufferers and 2% of the population. The occurrence of repeated thrombotic events (arterial and venous), including miscarriages and transient ischaemic attacks (TIAs), as well as cases of thrombosis at unusual sites, including cerebral or mesen-teric circulations, should highlight the possibility of antiphospholipid syn-drome. The first-line treatment is low-dose aspirin, but those with major thrombotic events such as a deep vein thrombosis (DVT) will often require anticoagulation with warfarin.

48. Medications in hyperkalaemia

E. Spironolactone

Amlodipine is a calcium channel blocker commonly used in hyperten-sion and does not affect serum potassium. Bendroflumethiazide is a thia-zide diuretic and is known to lower serum potassium. Whilst it is largely ineffective at lowering blood pressure in renal failure, it may be reducing the serum potassium and so shouldn't be stopped. Furosemide is a loop diuretic, which also lowers serum potassium. If this man has come in with acute renal failure caused by hypovolaemia, furosemide should probably be stopped. Simvastatin is a statin and does not affect serum potassium. Spironolactone is an aldosterone antagonist and will increase the serum potassium, and for this reason, it should be stopped in renal failure, especially here, where the potassium level is raised. A serum potassium level of 5.5 mmol/L is not too high, but it should be checked that potassium is not being added to the patient's fluid prescription, as well as confirming that he is asymptomatic and checking his electrocardiogram (ECG) for changes.

49. Tumour markers

A. CA 125

The most concerning diagnosis in this case is ovarian carcinoma, for which CA 125 is a tumour marker. The clinical features of ovarian malignancy include weight loss, abdominal pain, increasing abdominal girth and ascites. Unfortunately, the symptoms of ovarian malignancy usually occur late, meaning the disease is often advanced and metastatic at presentation. Diagnosis usually involves ultrasound scanning, computed tomography (CT) imaging, ovarian biopsy and measurement of CA 125. Both chemotherapy and surgery have a role in the management of ovarian cancer and have both curative and palliative roles. Radiotherapy is now limited to the palliation of symptoms. Because ovarian malignancy usually presents late, the prognosis is poor. However, if the disease is diagnosed early and treated appropriately, survival rates for early-stage disease can be as high as 95% at 5 years.

Other examples of tumour markers are provided in the following table:

Alpha-fetoprotein	Hepatocellular carcinoma, germ cell tumours
Beta-hCG	Choriocarcinoma, testicular tumours
Ca 15-3	Breast cancer
Ca 19-9	Pancreatic cancer
Calcitonin	Medullary thyroid cancer
Carcinoembryonic antigen	Colorectal tumours
Monoclonal IgG (paraprotein)	Multiple myeloma
Neurone-specific enolase	Small cell lung cancer
Placental alkaline phosphatase	Ovarian carcinoma, testicular tumours
Prostate-specific antigen	Prostate cancer
S-100	Malignant melanoma
Thyroglobulin	Thyroid tumours

50. Parkinson's disease

D. Bradykinesia, postural instability, rigidity and tremor ~3–4 Hz

Parkinson's disease symptoms are mainly caused by a lack of dopamine in the basal ganglia, secondary to a loss of midbrain substantia nigra pars compacta neurones. Models of basal ganglia function suggest that they take inputs concerning "motor plans" from the motor and cognitive frontal cortex and then the dopamine acts as a gate to allow those motor plans to be executed. Hence, bradykinesia is a prominent symptom and is mostly related to the loss of dopamine. Postural instability appears late in the disease and may be seen as a lack of ability to voluntarily adjust position in response to postural disturbance. Rigidity is classically either "lead pipe" (stiff throughout range of movement) or "cogwheel" (essentially, lead-pipe rigidity with the tremor superimposed). The tremor of Parkinson's disease is the most common feature and is usually unilateral and about 3–4 Hz in frequency. It may take the form of the classic "pill-rolling" tremor. A tremor of 10–12 Hz seems too fast for Parkinson's disease, and other causes such as familial or essential tremor should be considered. Postural hypotension may occur but is more commonly a side effect of levodopa (L-DOPA) therapy or associated with the "Parkinson-plus" syndrome, which is multiple system atrophy. Micrographia (small writing) and mask-like facies are also features of Parkinson's disease but are less important diagnostically and functionally than the four main features.

James Parkinson, English surgeon (1755-1824)

Practice paper 4: Questions

1. Airway management

You find an 80-year-old man collapsed in the street. He is unresponsive and is making a snoring sound. An ambulance has been called but has yet to arrive.

Which of the following is the best course of action?

A Cricothyroidotomy
B Do nothing until the ambulance arrives
C Finger sweep
D Head tilt–chin lift
E Place in the recovery position

2. Management of pulmonary embolism

A 26-year-old woman presents to the emergency department with a 1-week history of increased breathlessness on exertion. Her oxygen saturation is 80% on room air. She has not travelled abroad recently and does not have a family history of thromboembolism. On examination, the jugular venous pressure is elevated, and there is an accentuation of the pulmonary component of the second heart sound. The chest examination is unremarkable. A chest X-ray is normal. A subsequent CT pulmonary angiogram demonstrated a pulmonary embolism.

Which of the following management techniques is NOT appropriate?

A Request an echocardiogram
B Request a thrombophilia screen
C Request tumour markers
D Start treatment with low-molecular-weight heparin
E Start warfarin treatment

3. Skin manifestations of systemic disease

A 34-year-old woman presents to the GP complaining of a new rash. The skin under her arms and on the back of her neck is dark and velvety in texture. She has a past medical history of diabetes for which she takes insulin.

DOI: 10.1201/9781003648222-7

What is the most likely diagnosis?

A Acanthosis nigricans
B Diabetic dermopathy
C Erythema ab igne
D Hyperhidrosis
E Xanthelasma

4. Scoring systems

Which of the following scoring systems can be used to assess the risk of an adverse outcome following an upper gastrointestinal bleed?

A Breslow score
B CURB-65 (Confusion, Urea, Respiratory rate, Blood pressure, Age) score
C Ranson's criteria
D Rockall score
E Waterlow score

5. Diagnosis of abdominal pain

A 64-year-old man presents to the emergency department with a large rectal bleed and left-sided abdominal pain. He has a long history of constipation. He is pyrexial at 38.4°C, and his heart rate is 110 bpm.

What is the most likely cause?

A Angiodysplasia
B Bowel malignancy
C Diverticulitis
D Haemorrhoids
E Pseudomembranous colitis

6. Investigation of hepatomegaly

A 55-year-old man is being investigated for an irregular heart rhythm. He has a past medical history of diabetes mellitus. He explains that exercise is difficult for him due to joint pains. During the examination it is noted that he is tanned in appearance and has hepatomegaly.

Which of the following investigations could reveal the aetiology of his symptoms?

A Haematinics
B Serum caeruloplasmin
C Short Synacthen test
D Alpha-1 antitrypsin
E Gamma-GT

7. Substance use

A 64-year-old woman is an inpatient on a surgical ward following an above-knee amputation. The nursing staff said she vomited earlier, and she has been unresponsive since her operation a few hours ago. On examination, you noticed her pupils are small and she has a respiratory rate of 5 breaths/min.

Which of the following is the most likely reason for this clinical picture?

A Alcohol withdrawal
B Opiate use
C Opiate withdrawal
D Sedative use
E Sedative withdrawal

8. Home oxygen

A 66-year-old man with a 10-year history of chronic obstructive pulmonary disease (COPD) is assessed in the respiratory clinic for eligibility for long-term domiciliary oxygen therapy.

Which of the following is NOT a criterion for prescription of long-term oxygen therapy?

A No exacerbation of COPD for the previous 5 weeks
B Patient has stopped smoking
C Patient has chronic hypoxaemia with $PaO_2 < 7.3$ kPa
D Presence of pulmonary hypertension with $PaO_2 < 8.0$ kPa
E Two arterial blood gases showing $PaO_2 < 7.3$ kPa within 7 days

9. Management of chest pain

Recently, a 68-year-old woman has not been coping at home. She is now experiencing episodes of central, heavy chest pain and shortness of breath on exertion. Her ECG is normal, as are her bloods and chest X-ray.

Which of the following will NOT help her during her next episode?

A Bisoprolol
B Glyceryl trinitrate (GTN) spray
C Rest
D Oxygen
E Salbutamol nebulisers

10. Antibiotics in pregnancy

A 33-year-old woman who is 10 weeks' pregnant develops increased frequency of urination and dysuria. Urine dip is positive for nitrites.

Which of the following antibiotics could be used to empirically treat the urinary tract infection?

A Ciprofloxacin
B Co-amoxiclav
C Doxycycline
D Trimethoprim
E Vancomycin

11. Left ventricular hypertrophy

An 80-year-old man attends the general practice for an annual check-up of his hypertension. He tells you about his "left ventricular hyper-thingummy". You check him and his records for confirmatory signs and symptoms.

Which of the following is NOT a sign of left ventricular hypertrophy?

A Inverted T-waves
B Left axis deviation
C Pansystolic murmur
D R-wave in V6 > 25 mm
E The sum of the magnitude of the S-wave in V1 and R-wave in V5 > 35 mm

12. Shortness of breath

A 79-year-old woman who was admitted to hospital with a fractured right neck of the femur 1 week ago suddenly becomes acutely unwell on the ward 6 days after her operation. She complains of sudden onset of shortness of breath and chest tightness. The pain is exacerbated by deep breathing. She has a past medical history of hypertension, hypercholesterolaemia and asthma. Her observations include temperature 37.8°C, pulse rate 108 bpm, blood pressure 96/66 mmHg, respiratory rate 26/min and O_2 saturations of 89% on room air. On examination, her chest is clear to both auscultation and percussion. An electrocardiogram (ECG) shows sinus tachycardia without bundle branch block.

What is the most likely diagnosis?

A Acute exacerbation of asthma
B Myocardial infarction
C Pneumonia
D Pneumothorax
E Pulmonary embolism (PE)

13. Polycystic kidney disease

A 43-year-old man presents with intermittent haematuria. On exam of the abdomen, bilateral masses are felt, and an ultrasound reveals polycystic kidneys. You explain the syndrome to him. He is concerned that his son may develop the disease and doesn't believe his wife suffers from the condition.

What is the probability that his son will develop the disease?

A Negligible

B One in two

C One in four

D One in a thousand

E One in two thousand

14. Management of status epilepticus

A 35-year-old homeless man presents to the emergency department unconscious and has been for 35 minutes. He smells of alcohol and looks dishevelled. He has an adequate airway and requires oxygen therapy in the form of 10 L/min. His pulse and blood pressure are within normal range, and capillary glucose is normal. What should his immediate management be?

A Diazepam 2 mg intravenously

B Diazepam 2 mg intravenously and Pabrinex intravenously

C Lorazepam 4 mg intravenously and Pabrinex intravenously

D Lorazepam 8 mg intravenously

E Lorazepam 8 mg intravenously and Pabrinex intravenously

15. Overdose and antidotes

A 17-year-old female took 20 paracetamol tablets 3 hours ago in an attempt to end her life after an argument with her mum. She has now attended hospital with regret and is asking for treatment.

Which of the following should be administered?

A Atropine

B Desferrioxamine

C Digibind

D *N*-acetylcysteine

E Sodium bicarbonate

16. Murmur

You are examining a tearful young child who has fractured her arm. On auscultation you hear an ejection systolic murmur. There is no cyanosis.

Which of the following prevents you from reassuring her calm dad that his daughter has no serious heart problem?

A A history of cyanosis

B The fracture needs to heal first

C The second heart sound is split

D The murmur disappears on sitting up

E The murmur is soft

17. Management of shortness of breath

A 60-year-old man presents to the emergency department with shortness of breath for 3 hours and chest pain. He also complains of a right calf pain that he has had for 2 weeks. He has a past medical history of hypertension, recent stroke and disseminated lung cancer. His observations include temperature 37.0°C, pulse rate 112 bpm, blood pressure 100/54 mmHg, respiratory rate 26/min and saturations 87% on room air. There is no significant finding on chest examination. An electrocardiogram (ECG) shows sinus tachycardia and new right bundle branch block. A computed tomography (CT) pulmonary angiography confirmed massive pulmonary embolism.

What is the most appropriate initial treatment?

A Intravenous caval filters
B Oral warfarin
C Prophylactic dose of low-molecular-weight heparin
D Thrombolysis
E Treatment dose of low-molecular-weight heparin

18. *Helicobacter pylori* infection

A 55-year-old man is found to have a gastric ulcer following an endoscopy for left upper quadrant pain. A rapid urease test is positive for *Helicobacter pylori* infection.

What treatment does this man need?

A H_2 antagonist plus metronidazole and clarithromycin
B Metronidazole, clarithromycin and amoxicillin
C PPI plus metronidazole and clarithromycin
D PPI plus H_2 antagonist plus an antibiotic
E Steroids plus PPI plus metronidazole

19. Management of hyperglycaemia

A 55-year-old man presents to his GP with increasing lethargy and polyuria. He has a past medical history of ischaemic heart disease and congestive cardiac failure. He smokes 30 cigarettes per day and drinks alcohol occasionally. He has a body mass index (BMI) of 32 kg/m². His random blood glucose is 14.0 mmol/L and fasting blood glucose level is 9.0 mmol/L.

Which of the following management options is NOT appropriate in this patient?

A Advise the patient to change his diet and stop smoking
B Metformin should be considered as the first-line oral treatment option for overweight patients
C Sulphonylureas and metformin could be considered as a combined therapy if glycaemic control is not optimal
D Sulphonylureas should be considered if patient is intolerant to metformin
E Thiazolidinediones can be added to metformin and sulphonylurea combination therapy if control is not optimal

20. Drug administration

A 79-year-old woman is started on high-dose steroids for giant cell arteritis. As therapy will likely be maintained for at least a year, she needs bone protection. The decision is made to start alendronate 70 mg once weekly.

How would you advise her to take the tablet?

A Take it in bed at least half an hour before rising for breakfast
B Take it whilst sitting or standing just before breakfast
C Take it whilst sitting or standing upright at least half an hour after breakfast with minimal sips of water
D Take it with plenty of water whilst sitting or standing upright at least half an hour after breakfast
E Take it whilst sitting or standing upright at least half an hour before breakfast with plenty of water

21. Arterial blood gases

A 59-year-old man is admitted to the emergency department following a fall. He complains of increased tiredness and jerking movement of his legs, which led to his fall from the staircase. He is a smoker. On arrival, he has an oxygen saturation level of 76% in air, and an arterial blood gas reading demonstrates pH 7.40, PaO_2 6 kPa, $PaCO_2$ 9.3 kPa and HCO_3^- 35 mEq/L on room air (reference ranges: pH 7.35–7.45, PaO_2 11–13 kPa, $PaCO_2$ 4.7–6.0 kPa, HCO_3^- 22–26 mEq/L). His respiratory rate was 20/min.

What does this blood gas result show?

A Acute type 1 respiratory failure
B Acute type 2 respiratory failure
C Compensated chronic type 2 respiratory failure
D Metabolic acidosis
E Respiratory alkalosis

22. Fluid therapy

A 55-year-old man fractures his ankle attempting to replicate the latest dance fad he has seen his children do. He is otherwise well and is haemodynamically stable. The fracture requires open reduction and internal fixation. The trauma registrar has said that he needs to be kept nil by mouth from midnight; however, the operating list is always changing, and new emergencies may come in. There are at least three cases that are likely to get done before him. Your request that he have breakfast, as he is likely to be done later in the day is met with derision. He will need physiological fluid replacement when he is nil by mouth. He weighs 70 kg.

Which of the following regimens is closest to physiological needs?

A 1 L 0.9% normal saline with 20 mmol potassium and 2 × 1 L 5% dextrose in 24 hours

B 1 L 0.9% normal saline with 20 mmol potassium and 2 × 1 L 5% dextrose with 20 mmol potassium in 24 hours

C 2 × 1 L 0.9% normal saline with 20 mmol potassium and 1 L 5% dextrose in 24 hours

D 2 × 1 L 0.9% normal saline with 20 mmol potassium and 1 L 5% dextrose with 20 mmol potassium in 24 hours

E 3 L Hartmann's in 24 hours

23. Haemolytic anaemia

In haemolytic anaemia which is the correct pattern of investigations that you would expect to see?

A Low haemoglobin, low unconjugated bilirubin, high haptoglobin

B Low haemoglobin, high unconjugated bilirubin, high urinary urobilinogen, low haptoglobin

C Microcytic anaemia, normal bilirubin, high transferrin, low ferritin

D Normocytic anaemia, normal bilirubin, low iron, low TIBC, normal ferritin

E Normal haemoglobin, raised conjugated bilirubin, normal haptoglobin

24. Basic life support

You are the designated driver on Saturday night and are soberly walking to your car with your friends. You spot an elderly man lying on the ground. He is not breathing and has no pulse, although he is warm. You ask a friend to call 999. His airway is clear. Your precordial thump fails.

The most likely way for his heart to resume beating is:

A Adrenaline

B Defibrillation

C Cerebral reoxygenation

D Chest compressions

E Recovery position

25. Causes of tremor

Which of the following diseases is the most common reason for misdiagnosis of Parkinson's disease?

A Corticobasal degeneration
B Essential tremor/familial tremor
C Progressive supranuclear palsy
D Pugilist encephalopathy
E Wilson's disease

26. Biological therapies

A 46-year-old woman has been diagnosed with rheumatoid arthritis and has been on methotrexate for over a year, but sadly her disease is not under control. She wants to know about the new drugs used for rheumatoid arthritis that she heard about at a patients' association.

Which of the following statements about biological disease-modifying antirheumatic drugs (DMARDs) is NOT true?

A A chest X-ray should be taken before starting to rule out latent tuberculosis (which could be reactivated)
B If the patient's disease gets worse whilst on biological therapy, switching from one biological DMARD to another is unlikely to produce an improvement
C Injection site reactions for subcutaneously injected agents are common
D The more commonly used agents target and inhibit tumour necrosis factor alpha (TNF-alpha)
E They can be used in combination with methotrexate

27. Cognitive impairment

A 55-year-old woman presents with mild cognitive impairment and disinhibition without significant mood change. She also has falls and urinary incontinence. She has no major past medical history or medications and has never smoked or drank much alcohol. On examination, there are no cranial nerve or arm defects; however, the legs appear to have increased tone, upgoing plantars and clonus bilaterally, with some weakness of hip and knee flexion bilaterally.

Which of the following diagnoses may explain the picture?

A Alzheimer's disease
B Benign intracranial hypertension
C Lewy body dementia
D Normal pressure hydrocephalus (NPH)
E Vascular dementia

28. Complications of blood transfusion

A 45-year-old man is having his second transfusion following blood loss from a road traffic collision. During the transfusion he developed a fever of 38.5°C and rigors.

What should your immediate action be?

A Contact haematology for urgent advice
B Give steroids and antihistamines and continue transfusion
C Start antibiotics
D Stop the transfusion, take blood cultures and provide supportive measures
E Take blood cultures and continue transfusion

29. Diagnosis of numbness

A 32-year-old woman presents to her GP complaining of tingling and numbness around her mouth for 1 week. Occasionally, she also develops painful carpal spasm. She has a past medical history of Graves' disease for which she just recently had subtotal thyroidectomy.

What is the most likely diagnosis?

A Hypercalcaemia
B Hypermagnesaemia
C Hypocalcaemia
D Hypophosphataemia
E Hypothyroidism

30. Diagnosis of postural hypotension

A 62-year-old woman presents to the emergency department with collapse. She felt dizzy when she tried to stand up from a sitting position. She did not lose consciousness. She denied any visual disturbances, headache or head injury. She also complained of fatigue over the past month. She takes only omeprazole and paracetamol. An ECG showed normal sinus rhythm. Blood pressure was 102/50 mmHg with a postural systolic drop of 30 mmHg. Blood test revealed Na^+ 126 mmol/L, K^+ 6.5 mmol/L, urea 10.0 mmol/L and creatinine 139 µmol/L.

Which of the following will be most useful in establishing the diagnosis?

A Low-dose dexamethasone suppression test
B Random cortisol level
C Renal ultrasound scan
D Short Synacthen test
E Water deprivation test

31. Management of delirium

A 70-year-old man admitted 2 days previously with a mechanical fall and needing rehabilitation becomes increasingly anxious and agitated on the ward. He has been pestering the nurses for some "moonshine", and he is now disorientated in place and time. He claims to have seen little gnomes dashing between patients' beds. You suspect delirium tremens.

Which of the following represents the best management?

A Intravenous Pabrinex
B Oral Pabrinex
C Reducing the dose of chlordiazepoxide
D Reducing the dose of chlordiazepoxide and intravenous Pabrinex
E Reducing the dose of chlordiazepoxide and oral Pabrinex

32. Liver function tests

Which of the following results is the best indicator of poor liver function?

A Raised alanine transferase
B Raised albumin
C Raised alkaline phosphatase
D Raised bilirubin
E Prolonged prothrombin time

33. Diagnosis of cough

A 60-year-old woman presents to her GP with a chronic cough associated with thick, yellow sputum for the past year. Sometimes, the sputum is blood tinged. She had been prescribed multiple courses of antibiotics, but they did not seem to help. She has a past medical history of severe pneumonia that required admission to the intensive care unit for 20 days. On chest examination, there are inspiratory crackles throughout the lung fields, with normal vesicular breath sounds.

Which of the following is the most likely differential diagnosis?

A Bronchial carcinoma
B Bronchiectasis
C Chronic pulmonary obstructive disease
D Idiopathic pulmonary fibrosis
E Pneumonia

34. Diagnosis of skin lesions

A 31-year-old man presents with a 1-month history of a growing round, flat, erythematous lesion on the left thigh. The border is slightly more erythematous than the rest of the lesion and has some flakiness of the skin. The lesion itches. The patient also has had long-standing itchy scales between his toes.

Which of the following investigations would help confirm the most likely diagnosis?

A Excisional biopsy
B Incisional biopsy
C Punch biopsy
D Skin scrapings to be sent for microscopy culture and sensitivities
E Skin swab to be sent for microscopy culture and sensitivities

35. Electrocardiogram

A 56-year-old man has a myocardial infarction the day after a hernia repair. You request an ECG and then compare it to his pre-admission trace. You notice ST-segment changes in leads II, III and aVF.

In which part of the myocardium is the infarct?

A Anterior
B Anterolateral
C Anteroseptal
D Inferior
E Posterior

36. Diagnosis of neurological dysfunction

A 19-year-old female university student presents with problems in both arms and difficulty walking. Since starting her course, she has had difficulty writing, typing and other such activities and thus has struggled to keep up with the workload. She says the arms have "felt unusual" for around 6 months. She describes finding small burns and blisters on her arms that she can't remember getting in the first place. In the last few weeks, she has also fallen twice when walking up the stairs. The only other thing she describes is some mild occipital headaches that have increased in frequency lately. She is otherwise fit and well.

On examination, there is a loss of pinprick sensation found throughout the arms and on the back to around the T3 level. Her hands appear to have some element of small muscle wasting, and there is some loss of power throughout the arms. Reflexes are hard to elicit or possibly absent. In the legs, there is some mild symmetrical weakness, and the knee reflexes appear brisk. Plantars appear equivocal.

What is the most likely diagnosis?

A Cervical spondylosis
B Multiple sclerosis
C Psychogenic neurological symptoms
D Syringomyelia
E Viral transverse myelitis

37. Management of ischaemic stroke

A 74-year-old woman presents to hospital with an acute right-sided hemiparesis and is found to have a left middle cerebral artery infarct on diffusion-weighted magnetic resonance imaging (MRI). It is her first stroke. Her past medical history is unremarkable. Her blood pressure is normal, and her electrocardiogram (ECG) shows sinus rhythm with occasional ventricular ectopics. Blood tests show normal cholesterol and normal glucose. On carotid Doppler she is found to have an 85% stenosis of the left carotid artery.

Which of the following treatments will NOT benefit her?

A ACE inhibitor
B Aspirin
C Left carotid endarterectomy
D Statin
E Warfarin

38. Malignant melanoma

A 24-year-old woman who has been travelling to India on a gap year presents to clinic, as she is concerned about a "funny-looking mole" on her leg. She is unsure how long it has been there.

Which of the following is NOT a concerning feature of a mole when considering a diagnosis of malignant melanoma?

A Asymmetry
B Bleeding
C Border irregularity
D Colour different from that of other moles on the patient
E Itching

39. Nipple discharge

A 42-year-old woman presents to her GP with a 2-month history of nipple discharge from her left breast. The discharge is milky in colour. No blood is noted. She has a medical history of hypertension, type 2 diabetes mellitus and depression. She has been taking regular medication for these conditions. She has been amenorrhoeic for 6 months. A provisional diagnosis of hyperprolactinaemia is made.

What of the following is NOT appropriate management?

A Breast examination
B Serum prolactin
C Stop antidepressants
D Thyroid function tests
E Urgent computed tomography (CT) of the brain

40. Palpitations

A 52-year-old woman presents to the GP with intermittent palpitations and breathlessness that has occurred over the last few weeks. She denies chest pain. Her electrocardiogram (ECG) shows sinus tachycardia, and she does not appear to be anaemic.

Which blood test would be of most use in confirming the diagnosis?

A Haematinics
B Lactate
C No blood test required
D Thyroid function tests
E Troponin

41. Diagnosis of endocrine disease

A 33-year-old man presents to his GP complaining of worsening headaches and tiredness for the last 2 months. He denies drinking alcohol and smokes occasionally. He has a good appetite and has gained 3 pounds over the past month. He also noticed that he has difficulty in biting his food and has a reduced libido. On examination, he is tall, with an oval-shaped face, large hands and prominent lower jaw.

Which of the following tests is the most diagnostic in the initial diagnosis?

A Growth hormone levels during an oral glucose tolerance test
B IGF-1 levels
C MRI scan of pituitary fossa
D Pituitary function test
E Random growth hormone levels

42. Emollient use

In which of the following circumstances would use of emollients be ill-advised?

A Acne vulgaris
B Contact dermatitis
C Eczema
D Psoriasis
E Wound healing

43. Medications in acute renal failure

An 83-year-old man is admitted with acute confusion. He has an extensive medical history including atrial fibrillation, type 2 diabetes, osteoarthritis, hypertension and some mild congestive cardiac failure, for which he takes several medications. He appears clinically dry, with a pulse of 115/min, dry mucous membranes and a capillary refill rate of 4 seconds. He is noted to have a reduced urine output with concentrated urine. His creatinine is 235 μmol/L.

Which of the following medications does NOT need be reduced or stopped?

A Amlodipine
B Diclofenac
C Digoxin

D Furosemide
E Metformin

44. Rectal bleeding

A 27-year-old woman presents to the GP complaining of intense sharp pain on passing stools, accompanied by bright red bleeding noticed on the toilet paper. She has no fever and is otherwise well in herself. She recently had a course of codeine phosphate following a sprain injury to her ankle.

What is the most likely diagnosis?

A Anal abscess
B Anal carcinoma
C Anal fissure

D Crohn's disease
E Haemorrhoids

45. Signs of liver disease

A 15-year-old girl is being investigated for behavioural changes and is found to have a green-yellow discolouration around her iris on slit lamp examination.

What is the name of this feature?

A Arcus senilis
B Caput medusae
C Kayser–Fleischer rings

D Lens dislocation
E Xanthoma

46. Indications for haemodialysis in acute renal failure

Which of the following is NOT an indication for haemodialysis in patients with acute renal failure?

A Acidosis with a pH < 7.2
B Hypertension > 220 mmHg systolic or 160 mmHg diastolic
C Persistent potassium of > 7 mmol/L
D Refractory pulmonary oedema
E Uraemic pericarditis

47. Sexually transmitted infections

A 43-year-old woman attends the GP with a 3-month history of a grey-white vaginal discharge, which she says has a "fishy" odour. She is systemically well and has no menstrual abnormalities.

What is the most likely diagnosis?

A Bacterial vaginosis (BV)
B *Candida*
C Chlamydia

D Gonorrhoea
E Syphilis

48. Systemic lupus erythematosus

A 35-year-old woman has had a diffuse mild arthralgia with a fluctuating time course for the last year. There is never much synovitis to be seen on examination, and inflammatory markers are only mildly raised. ANA is positive.

Which of the following would make a diagnosis of systemic lupus erythematosus (SLE)?

A Anterior uveitis
B Anti-ribonucleoprotein antibodies
C Erosions on X-rays of affected joints
D Painful, palpable, purple lumps on the shins
E Red rash across the cheeks that is worse in summer

49. Uraemia

Which of the following is NOT a sign of uraemia?

A Clouding of consciousness   D Spider naevi
B Hiccoughs   E Twitching
C Lemon-yellow skin tone

50. Urinary frequency

A 30-year-old man presents to the medical assessment unit with a history of excessive drinking and urination. He has been going to the toilet about seven to eight times per day for 1 month. His random blood glucose is 9.3 mmol. His results on admission show:

Na⁺	147 mmol/L
K+	3.5 mmol/L
Urea	2.4 mmol/L
Creatinine	80 µmol/L
Corrected Ca²⁺	2.34 mmol/L
Plasma osmolality	609 mOsm/kg
Urine osmolality	145 mOsm/kg

(Peak osmolality pre-DDAVP reached 150 mOSm)

Water deprivation test – urine osmolality 600 mOsm/kg after DDAVP 2 µg administered intramuscularly

What is the most likely diagnosis?

A Acute tubular necrosis
B AVP deficiency (cranial diabetes insipidus)
C AVP resistance (nephrogenic diabetes insipidus)
D Primary polydipsia
E Type 2 diabetes mellitus

Practice paper 4: Answers

1. Airway management

D. Head tilt–chin lift

The head tilt and chin lift is the airway manoeuvre of choice when cervical spine trauma is not suspected. To achieve this, the patient is placed on their back, and the rescuer simultaneously lifts the patient's chin whilst extending the patient's head. This simple manoeuvre lifts the collapsed soft tissues and restores airway patency. Once the manoeuvre has been completed, the rescuer can reassess the airway by looking for chest movement and feeling for the patient's breath on their cheek. If the airway is patent and the patient is breathing spontaneously, they can be placed in the recovery position. If the patient is not breathing, basic life support measures should commence. The jaw thrust manoeuvre is the preferred choice when cervical spine trauma is suspected.

2. Management of pulmonary embolism

C. Request tumour markers

The examination findings suggest the presence of pulmonary hypertension. Therefore a transthoracic echocardiography could provide possible findings of right heart dilatation and a non-invasive assessment of pulmonary artery pressure. Thrombophilia screening should be considered in these patients with no known increased risk of venous thromboembolism. A treatment dose of low-molecular-weight heparin and warfarin are standard therapy for patients with diagnosed pulmonary embolism.

3. Skin manifestations of systemic disease

A. Acanthosis nigricans

The presence of a thickened, dark, velvety overgrowth in the axillae, neck and groin is typical of acanthosis nigricans. This rash is associated with insulin resistance (diabetes), Cushing's syndrome, acromegaly, polycystic ovarian syndrome, lymphomas and adenocarcinomas of the gastrointestinal tract.

Other cutaneous features of internal malignancy include Paget's disease (scaly, eczematous rash on the nipple – breast cancer); thrombophlebitis

DOI: 10.1201/9781003648222-8

migrans (recurrent thrombophlebitis in different parts of the body – pancreatic cancer); tylosis (hyperkeratosis of the palm and soles – oesophageal cancer); dermatomyositis (purple rash on eyelids and scaly pink rash on knuckles – lung and breast cancer); and necrolytic migratory erythema (blistering erythematous rash of buttocks, groin and legs – glucagonoma).

Diabetic dermopathy describes the presence of depressed pigmented scars in the shin. It is associated with diabetic microangiopathy. Other skin features of diabetes include necrobiosis lipoidica diabeticorum (shiny, atrophic yellowish–red plaques on the shins); cheiroarthropathy (a scleroderma-like thickening of the skin of the hands with limited joint mobility in insulin-dependent diabetics); granuloma annulare (small, papular lesions arranged in a ring and found on the back of the hands or feet); and acanthosis nigricans.

Erythema ab igne is a brown, lacy rash seen on skin that has been exposed to heat for long periods of time. It classically develops in hypothyroid patients who are cold intolerant and therefore spend a lot of time in front of the fire. Excessive hot water bottle use can also result in the rash. Hyperhidrosis is a condition involving excessive sweating. Xanthelasma are yellowish plaques around the eyelid and may be due to hyperlipidaemia.

Acanthosis nigricans, from Latin *acanthosis* = thorn + *neger* = black

Ab igne, from Latin *ab* = from + *ignis* = fire

4. Scoring systems

D. Rockall score

This scoring system can be used to predict adverse outcome following upper gastrointestinal bleeds by combining a number of independent risk factors (see the table). A score of >8 indicates a 40% risk of mortality.

Factor	0	1	2	3
Age	<60	60–79	>80	
Shock	BP >100 mmHg, pulse <100	BP >100 mmHg, pulse >100	BP <100 mmHg	
Co-morbidities	None	IHD, cardiac failure	Renal/liver failure	Metastatic malignancy
Diagnosis	Mallory–Weiss tear	All other except malignancy	Upper gastrointestinal malignancy	
Endoscopy	None		Active bleeding, adherent clot, visible vessels	

Rockall *et al*. Risk assessment after acute upper gastrointestinal haemorrhage. *Gut* 1996; 38:316–321.

The Breslow score is used as a prognostic factor in melanoma. Ranson's criteria helps to predict prognosis and mortality risk in acute pancreatitis. Waterlow score provides an estimated risk for developing a pressure sore in a patient. CURB-65 score estimates the mortality risk of a patient from community-acquired pneumonia.

5. Diagnosis of abdominal pain

C. Diverticulitis

A diverticulum is an out-pouching of a hollow structure. Colonic diverticula are examples of false diverticula – the walls are made up only of the inner mucosal layer of the bowel. A true diverticulum involves all the layers of the wall from which it arises, e.g. Meckel diverticulum. Diverticulosis describes the presence of colonic diverticula. Diverticular disease is a term used if complications arise from diverticulosis. Finally, diverticulitis specifically describes inflammation of the diverticula.

Colonic diverticula are most commonly found in the sigmoid and the descending colon. They are unusual in those under 40, but 30% of the elderly populations of developed countries are found to have diverticulosis at autopsy. The pathogenesis of diverticulosis is as follows: there is hypertrophy of the muscle of the sigmoid colon, resulting in high intraluminal pressures. This leads to herniation of the mucosa at potential sites of weakness in the bowel wall, which correspond to points of entry of blood vessels. The underlying aetiology of the initial large bowel hypertrophy is unknown, but it may be directly due to a diet that is chronically low in fibre. The diagnosis of diverticulosis is made by flexible sigmoidoscopy. A barium enema shows the diverticular out-pouching with a signet ring appearance due to filling defects produced by pellets of faeces within the diverticula. Complications of diverticulosis include lower gastrointestinal haemorrhage from erosion of a blood vessel within a diverticulum, obstruction from chronic diverticular infection and fibrosis and diverticulitis (infection of diverticula). In the acute phase of suspected diverticulitis, computed tomography (CT) is the best investigation. Treatment of diverticulitis is largely conservative: patients are kept nil by mouth with the administration of intravenous fluids and antibiotics until symptoms improve. Complications of diverticulitis include the formation of abscesses (which may perforate, leading to peritonitis), fistulae and strictures.

Angiodysplasia can present with a similar picture, although there is less of an inflammatory response and bleeding is usually painless. There are small hamartomas within the gut wall that are liable to bleed. This is less common than diverticular disease but may be diagnosed on endoscopy.

Pseudomembranous colitis is inflammation in the colon due to *Clostridium difficile*. This is commonly associated with antibiotic use.

Diverticulum, from Latin *di* = apart + *vertere* = to turn (i.e. a digression)

6. Investigation of hepatomegaly

A. Haematinics

The classical triad of haemochromatosis is bronze skin pigmentation, hepatomegaly and diabetes mellitus. Hereditary haemochromatosis is an autosomal recessive disease characterised by excess iron deposition in various organs throughout the body, which leads to their fibrosis and dysfunction. This question picks up on many of these complications: heart arrhythmias and possible heart failure and skin pigmentation due to iron deposition in the hypothalamus leading to excess melanin production and hypogonadism. Iron deposition in the liver leads to acute liver failure, whereas deposition in the pancreas leads to failure of its endocrine or exocrine function. Joints are generally affected in an asymmetrical fashion. Patients develop chondrocalcinosis due to development of calcium pyrophosphate crystals in the joint spaces. The diagnosis of haemochromatosis is made firstly from the haematinics, in which you would expect to see a raised ferritin, a reduced total iron binding capacity (due to saturation) and a transferrin saturation >60%. A liver biopsy will often show deposition of iron within the cells. The genetic loci for the common genes for haemochromatosis have also been located, with the two common mutations for the *HFE* gene being known. This can be useful in screening family members.

Addison's disease can result in a "tanned" skin appearance. It is due to primary adrenal failure caused by an autoimmune mechanism or tuberculosis. Short Synacthen test is the diagnostic test of choice in confirming Addison's disease.

7. Substance use

B. Opiate use

This patient is likely to be suffering the effects of opiate use. Examples of opiates include morphine, heroin, methadone and codeine. The effects of opiates, in addition to analgesia, include euphoria, nausea and vomiting, constipation, anorexia, hypotension, respiratory depression, tremor, pinpoint pupils and erectile dysfunction. The treatment of overdose (after completing an urgent airway, breathing and circulation [ABC] assessment) is with the antidote naloxone. This is ideally given intravenously but can be given intramuscularly or by inhalation. Depending on the doses required, an infusion of naloxone may be necessary, as the half-life is short. In contrast, the effects of opiate withdrawal can be extreme. They include dilated pupils, lacrimation, sweating, diarrhoea, insomnia, tachycardia, abdominal cramp-like pains, nausea and vomiting. Opiate dependence can be managed once drug use has stopped with methadone and buprenorphine (a partial agonist).

8. Home oxygen

E. Two arterial blood gases showing PaO$_2$ < 7.3 kPa within 7 days

Long-term domiciliary oxygen therapy is the provision of oxygen therapy for continuous use at home for patients with chronic hypoxaemia of PaO$_2$ at or below 7.3 kPa (55 mmHg) or nocturnal hypoventilation and for palliative use. Long-term domiciliary oxygen therapy can be prescribed in patients with chronic hypoxaemia with a PaO$_2$ between 7.3 and 8 kPa in the presence of pulmonary hypertension or secondary polycythaemia (haematocrit >55%). The aim of therapy is to increase the PaO$_2$ to at least 8 kPa (60 mmHg) or to attain saturations of at least 90%. Studies have shown long-term domiciliary oxygen therapy used for ≥15 hours/day in patients with COPD and chronic severe hypoxaemia improves survival, reduces secondary polycythaemia and prevents progression of primary pulmonary hypertension. For patients who are eligible for long-term oxygen therapy, three factors should be considered:

1. There should be a clinical diagnosis of a disorder associated with chronic hypoxaemia.
2. Patients should be on optimum medical treatment for a particular condition and clinically stable for at least 5 weeks.
3. Arterial blood gas tensions must be measured on two occasions not less than 3 weeks apart.

The patient should have stopped smoking and been made aware of the dangers of smoking in the presence of home oxygen therapy.

Refer to the British Thoracic Society guidelines on "Home oxygen use in adults": https://thorax.bmj.com/content/thoraxjnl/70/Suppl_1/i1.full.pdf

9. Management of chest pain

E. Salbutamol nebulisers

This woman has stable angina. GTN spray sublingually causes peripheral vasodilatation, reducing afterload and resting her myocardium. Oxygen will ensure that what blood is perfusing her myocardium is well oxygenated, minimizing hypoxia and its resultant anginal pain. Bisoprolol is a beta-blocker that will serve to cap the heart rate by blocking the beta-adrenergic receptors. Salbutamol nebulisers are not only of no benefit in this scenario (the patient does not have restricted airways) but also function as a beta-agonist, thus slightly stimulating the heart to work harder.

10. Antibiotics in pregnancy

B. Co-amoxiclav

This pregnant patient has a urinary tract infection (UTI) as evidenced by the presence of nitrites in urine dip. However, she has limited antibiotic treatment options available due to pregnancy. Ciprofloxacin, a quinolone antibiotic, is contraindicated in pregnancy, as animal studies have shown development of arthropathy in the child. Tetracyclines, such as doxycycline, bind calcium and thus become deposited in growing bones and teeth, limiting growth and staining teeth. Trimethoprim is a folate antagonist and thus carries a risk of teratogenicity. Vancomycin would have to be given intravenously, and this woman shows no indication of need for admission. This drug can cause severe side effects and so is reserved for dangerous or resistant organisms, and it has only Gram-positive cover, whereas 75% of community-acquired UTIs are caused by *Escherichia coli*, a Gram-negative organism. Co-amoxiclav provides good Gram-positive and Gram-negative cover and is commonly used in UTIs. Penicillins are not known to be harmful in pregnancy.

11. Left ventricular hypertrophy

C. Pansystolic murmur

The heart can face an increased afterload in aortic stenosis, hypertension and raised peripheral vascular resistance. In this "pressure overload" state, therefore, its response, like any muscle, is to develop increased bulk. A larger muscle radiates a larger depolarisation charge, manifesting in an increased QRS amplitude and left axis deviation. This creates two problems: (1) coronary arteries must traverse and support a thickened myocardium and (2) end-diastolic volume is reduced as the larger myocardium intrudes upon the ventricular chamber. This can lead to acute coronary syndrome, signs of which include T-wave inversion. A pansystolic murmur can be a sign of mitral regurgitation, which is associated with left ventricular dilatation (a "volume overload" state).

12. Shortness of breath

E. Pulmonary embolism (PE)

PE occurs in around 1% of all patients admitted to hospital and accounts for around 5% of in-hospital deaths. It usually arises from a venous thrombosis in the pelvis or legs. The clots break off and travel to the right side of heart via the venous system before lodging in the pulmonary circulation causing pulmonary circulation failure. The risk factors include any cause of immobility or hypercoagulability, e.g. recent surgery, long trips/flights pregnancy or postpartum, recent stroke or myocardial infarction, disseminated malignancy, thrombophilia and prolonged bed rest. A Wells score is used to assess the clinical probability of a pulmonary embolism:

Clinically suspected deep vein thrombosis (DVT)	3.0 points
Heart rate > 100 bpm	1.5 points
Immobilisation > 3 days/surgery last 4 weeks	1.5 points
History of DVT/PE	1.5 points
Haemoptysis	1.0 points
Malignancy (palliative or treated in last 6 months)	1.0 points
Alternative diagnosis less likely	3 points

A score of <4 means a PE is unlikely, so consider measuring a D-dimer to rule out PE. D-dimer has a good negative predictive value for PE.

A score of more than 4 means a PE is likely, so consider imaging (computed tomography [CT] pulmonary angiography).

Philip Wells, Contemporary Professor of Medicine, University of Ottawa

13. Polycystic kidney disease

B. One in two

The most common form of polycystic kidney disease has a prevalence of 1 in 1000 and is inherited in an autosomal dominant manner. Therefore, assuming that his wife does not suffer from the disease, the chance of his son being affected is 1 in 2. There is a rarer autosomal recessive form with a prevalence of 1 in 40,000.

14. Management of status epilepticus

C. Lorazepam 4 mg intravenously and Pabrinex intravenously

Diazepam or lorazepam can be used, but 2 mg of intravenous diazepam is too low a dose – 10 mg is the recommended dose. Lorazepam 4 mg should be used initially. If there is no effect after 5 minutes, a further 4 mg can be used. Intravenous Pabrinex (vitamin B complex) is being used in this case, as there is a possibility of alcohol withdrawal which, in the presence of B_1 deficiency (not unlikely in chronic alcoholism), can potentially cause Wernicke's encephalopathy (presenting with confusion, oculomotor dysfunction and ataxia), which may progress to irreversible Korsakoff syndrome – severe impairment of new memory formation, some impairment of accessing old memories and confabulation.

15. Overdose and antidotes

D. *N*-acetylcysteine

Paracetamol is widely available, cheap and extremely toxic in overdose. It is one of the most common drugs implicated in intentional overdose and is usually taken in combination with alcohol and/or other substances. There are usually no initial symptoms of paracetamol overdose, which often leads to the patient believing they have caused no harm. Late features of overdose include vomiting, abdominal pain, bruising, jaundice and encephalopathy. If a patient presents with paracetamol overdose, a serum paracetamol level should be tested at 4 hours after the overdose was taken in addition to a full blood count, liver function tests, serum glucose and a coagulation screen. When a therapeutic dose of paracetamol is taken, the hepatotoxic metabolites are conjugated with glutathione, which neutralises their toxicity. In paracetamol overdose the endogenous glutathione pathways become saturated, allowing the hepatotoxic metabolites to build up and cause hepatic necrosis. *N*-acetylcysteine is the first-line antidote in paracetamol overdose and works by restoring the levels of glutathione, which conjugates and neutralises the toxins. It should ideally be started within 8 hours of the patient taking the overdose but can be given up to 24 hours after the overdose. If a patient presents more than 24 hours after overdose, a specialist liver unit should be contacted for advice.

The decision to treat with *N*-acetylcysteine is usually based upon the serum paracetamol level taken at least 4 hours after the overdose. The paracetamol level is applied to a normogram that plots the time since overdose against the serum paracetamol level. On the normogram there is a "low-risk" treatment line and a "high-risk" treatment line. If the patient's paracetamol level is plotted above the treatment line, they will require *N*-acetylcysteine. If the patient is taking enzyme-inducing drugs or has pre-existing liver disease the "high-risk" treatment line should be used (which in practice means that this group is treated in the presence of lower serum paracetamol levels compared to patients who are not considered to be high risk). In cases of delayed presentation, extreme overdose, staggered overdose and unconsciousness, it is often appropriate to treat prior to taking a 4-hour paracetamol level. If the patient has had a prior allergic reaction to *N*-acetylcysteine, the alternative antidote is methionine.

16. Murmur

A. A history of cyanosis

Benign murmurs are common, especially in children. A Still murmur is a soft ejection systolic murmur that disappears on sitting up (it is benign). Young children require vigorous cardiac output through comparatively narrow vessels; this can lead to a pulmonary flow murmur. The increased pulmonary vein pressure can lead to a delay in pulmonary valve closure – a split second heart sound. In children, the jugular vein walls can vibrate with the comparatively brisk venous circulation; this is known as a "venous hum" and is also benign. Fractured arms do not cause heart problems other than by secondary hypovolaemia – and dad would not be calm if this was the case!

Ventricular septal defects are the most common congenital cardiac defect and may present as a soft pansystolic murmur. If large, corrective surgery will be indicated; large defects ultimately cause cyanosis as an initial left-right shunt leads to an increased pulmonary vascular resistance reversing the shunt (and ending the cyanosis) – Eisenmenger syndrome. This will become a life-threatening problem and needs to be corrected.

Sir George Still also gave his name to juvenile idiopathic arthritis (Still disease) and was the first doctor to document attention deficit hyperactivity disorder in his lectures of 1902.

Murmur, from Sanskrit *marmara* = rustling sound

Victor Eisenmenger, Austrian physician (1864-1932)

George Frederic Still, English paediatrician (1868-1941)

17. Management of shortness of breath

E. Treatment dose of low-molecular-weight heparin

If there is an acute massive pulmonary embolism that is accompanied by shock, thrombolytic therapy appears to improve outcome. However, in this case, the patient has high haemorrhagic risk, and thus, it is not appropriate to administer thrombolytic therapy (e.g. alteplase). Anticoagulation therapy with low-molecular-weight heparin is effective in reducing mortality in pulmonary embolism by reducing the propagation of clot and the risk of further emboli. It is administered for at least 5 days, and anticoagulation is commenced using oral warfarin.

18. *Helicobacter pylori* infection

C. PPI plus metronidazole and clarithromycin

H. pylori is a spiral-shaped, Gram-negative bacteria found to be a causative organism in the development of gastric ulcers. It is able to colonise the harshly acidic environment of the stomach due to a urease enzyme that can locally convert urea into ammonia (which neutralises the surrounding acid) and carbon dioxide. *H. pylori* causes gastritis by inciting an inflammatory response from the host. It is implicated in gastric and duodenal ulcers, as well as gastric carcinoma. There are several different tests available, including a C_{13} urea breath test, serological tests, tissue biopsy (rapid urease test, histology and culture) and stool test detecting antibodies to the bacterium. Eradication is via triple therapy (a proton pump inhibitor [PPI] such as omeprazole plus two relevant antibiotics) with a repeat endoscopy to show resolution of the ulcer. This treatment regimen is given for 14 days.

19. Management of hyperglycaemia

E. Thiazolidinediones can be added to metformin and sulphonylurea combination therapy if control is not optimal

Management of diabetes mellitus includes non-pharmacological and pharmacological treatments. Lifestyle changes such as regular exercise; having a healthy, balanced diet; and reducing alcohol consumption all could improve glycaemic control. The aim of pharmacological treatment in diabetes mellitus is to lower the blood glucose level, which will provide relief from symptoms such as polyuria and polydipsia and reduce the risks of micro- and macro-vascular complications. Metformin acts by decreasing hepatic gluconeogenesis and improves peripheral glucose uptake while suppressing appetite and promoting weight reduction. It should be considered the first-line oral treatment for patients with type 2 diabetes, especially when they are overweight. Sulphonylureas such as gliclazide and glipizide act by stimulating the release of insulin from pancreatic beta cells. They are considered in patients who do not tolerate metformin or in those in whom it is contraindicated. Metformin and a sulphonylurea could be considered as a combined therapy, as they act synergistically. Thiazolidinediones work by activating peroxisome proliferator-activated receptor-γ, which regulates the expression of several genes involving metabolism, and enhancing the actions of endogenous insulin. They are used as a third-line therapy in combination with metformin and sulphonylureas; however, they cause sodium and fluid retention and should not be used in patients with cardiac failure, such as in this case.

20. Drug administration

E. Take it whilst sitting or standing upright at least half an hour before breakfast with plenty of water

A dangerous side effect of alendronate (also known as alendronic acid) is that it can cause oesophagitis, oesophageal erosions, oesophageal ulcers and oesophageal strictures. To avoid this, the exposure of alendronate to the oesophagus should be minimised. First, alendronate should be avoided in disorders that delay oesophageal emptying (e.g. strictures) and used cautiously in patients with dysphagia or reflux. Secondly, it should be taken upright so that gravity reduces transit time and reflux. Thirdly, by taking at least half an hour before any food, the chances of any alendronate refluxing into the oesophagus are reduced further. Fourthly, taking with lots of water should wash the alendronate through the oesophagus as swiftly as possible.

Owing to the complexity and inconvenience of taking alendronate and frequent side effects ranging from dyspepsia to those mentioned earlier, there is often poor compliance. If a patient on alendronate develops dysphagia or other oesophageal symptoms, it should be stopped. Intravenous bisphosphonates, which can be given less frequently (e.g. annual zoledronate), can be considered and are arguably more convenient but are more expensive.

21. Arterial blood gases

C. Compensated chronic type 2 respiratory failure

A history of smoking suggests underlying chronic obstructive pulmonary disease. A $PaCO_2 > 6.0$ kPa with a low pO_2 indicates type 2 respiratory failure, which would lead to respiratory acidosis. The pH can be expected to be acidotic; however, in this case the pH is within the normal range and there is a high compensated bicarbonate level, which suggests chronicity, and compensated type 2 respiratory failure.

22. Fluid therapy

B. 1 L 0.9% normal saline with 20 mmol potassium and 2 × 1 L 5% dextrose with 20 mmol potassium in 24 hours

A man weighing 70 kg (average weight) requires 2.5–3 L of water a day, so all options are valid in volumatic terms. In terms of electrolytes, 140 mmol of sodium and 60–70 mmol of potassium are needed. A quantity of 1 L of normal saline contains 154 mmol of sodium. Hartmann's contains 131 mmol of sodium and 5 mmol of potassium, as well as chloride, calcium and lactate. Therefore 3 L of Hartmann's will give too much sodium and not enough potassium, which could lead to fluid retention and hypokalaemia, respectively. Therefore do not get caught out by the "Hartmann's is more physiological" trap. However, Hartmann's may be more appropriate where there has been fluid and electrolyte loss (for instance, diarrhoea and vomiting). A quantity of 1 L of normal saline over the day will meet the patient's sodium needs, so it is between option A and option B. Option A provides 20 mmol of potassium, and option B provides 60 mmol of potassium; therefore option B is the right answer.

23. Haemolytic anaemia

B. Low haemoglobin, high unconjugated bilirubin, high urinary urobilinogen, low haptoglobin

Haemolytic anaemia is a pre-hepatic cause of jaundice. Haemolytic anaemia occurs when there is a shortening of the red cell life span (normal red cell life span is 120 days), and biochemically this will present as an increase in the products of red cell destruction, as well as increased bone marrow cell production. There are many causes of haemolytic anaemia, either due to a cause within the red cell itself or within the vessel. Problems within the red cell can be with the membrane or with the production, such as sickle cell disease. Extrinsic causes can be divided into immune or non-immune causes. Haptoglobin binds free haemoglobin; therefore levels decrease where there is increased red cell breakdown. Other biochemical signs of haemolytic anaemia are raised lactase dehydrogenase (LDH) and raised reticulocytes.

24. Basic life support

B. Defibrillation

A precordial thump upon the chest is only likely to cardiovert if given within seconds of a cardiac arrest. Chest compressions will move blood from the lungs to the cerebrum. This will prevent tissue hypoxia, leading to infarction and therefore reduce morbidity should the patient become successfully resuscitated; however, they are unlikely to restore a pulse. Only defibrillation will start the heart beating again, although his airway should always be checked first as per the ABC protocol.

Praecordium, from Latin *prae* = in front of + *cordis* = heart

25. Causes of tremor

B. Essential tremor/familial tremor

The other four diseases actually cause genuine extrapyramidal symptoms and signs; however, essential/familial tremor is far more common. As tremor is the most widely known and usually the earliest sign of Parkinson's disease and essential/familial tremor can present in late middle age, frequent misdiagnosis is understandable. Essential and familial tremor are similar, except essential tremor has no family history. These tremors are absent at rest but appear on action, have a frequency of 6–12 Hz and a fine amplitude, are present throughout the range of movement and may be ameliorated by alcohol or beta-blockers. No other parkinsonian symptoms are present. The parkinsonian tremor is present at rest but diminishes with action, has a frequency of 3–7 Hz and a coarse amplitude and commonly affects the distal limbs asymmetrically. Importantly, essential/familial tremor is separate from cerebellar tremor, which increases in magnitude throughout the movement to be maximal on approaching target, is usually 4–6 Hz and is associated with other cerebellar signs.

Progressive supranuclear palsy combines parkinsonian symptoms with a supranuclear gaze palsy, most commonly and initially affecting downgaze. Wilson's disease is a disorder of copper metabolism leading to copper deposition throughout the body, most commonly in the liver (causing liver disease) and basal ganglia (causing parkinsonian and other extrapyramidal symptoms, e.g. dystonia), as well as in the iris (Kayser–Fleischer rings). Usual onset is in the 20s–30s. Pugilist encephalopathy is a parkinsonian syndrome resulting from repeated head trauma (a pugilist is a boxer). Corticobasal degeneration is an exceedingly rare syndrome with bradykinesia and an unstable posture with dystonias, alien limb phenomenon and apraxia (tremor is not a prominent feature).

26. Biological therapies

B. If the patient's disease gets worse whilst on biological therapy, switching from one biological DMARD to another is unlikely to produce an improvement

The relatively older biological DMARDs, which are less expensive (but still more expensive than traditional DMARDs) and have more long-term data and experience of use, target and block TNF-alpha, a key inflammatory cytokine. Etanercept is a humanised TNF-alpha receptor fused with IgG1, whereas adalimumab and infliximab are monoclonal antibodies to TNF-alpha. They can indeed reactivate latent tuberculosis, and so a chest X-ray should always be taken before starting therapy to rule this out. Etanercept and adalimumab are given by subcutaneous injection (patients are taught to self-inject), and injection site reactions are a relatively common side effect. They work well alone, but data suggests that they work better when used in combination with methotrexate. Other than the synergistic effect of using two DMARDs with different modes of action, it is thought that methotrexate may reduce formation of antibodies against the biological DMARDs themselves. Finally, switching between anti–TNF-alpha agents often can regain control of the disease.

27. Cognitive impairment

D. Normal pressure hydrocephalus (NPH)

Whilst falls and urinary incontinence can occur in Alzheimer's disease, these appear late in disease progression and do not fit with the patient's young age or mild cognitive impairment. Those with Lewy body dementia experience hallucinations as a prominent feature (which are not mentioned), and these commonly co-exist with parkinsonian movement symptoms. This woman seems to have pyramidal signs in the legs and no arm symptoms. Vascular dementia occurs with multiple strokes or transient ischaemic attacks (TIAs), which this woman does not have a history of or risk factors for. Benign intracranial hypertension does not commonly cause dementia and was mainly included to confuse, with its mention of intracranial pressure. It presents with headaches, visual disturbance (papilloedema, which would be absent with normal pressure) and sometimes cranial nerve VI palsies. It is associated with obesity, oral contraceptive pill use and use of tetracycline.

NPH commonly presents with the triad of dementia, gait disturbance and urinary incontinence. In NPH, cerebrospinal fluid (CSF) flow has been impeded, but compensatory mechanisms have prevented raised pressure. The lateral ventricles are prominently dilated, and these ventricles exert local pressure on certain brain areas to give the classic clinical picture. Pressure on the frontal lobes gives the dementia, and pressure on the medial side of the motor cortex and the pyramidal tract fibres causes incontinence and pyramidal leg weakness (remember the somatotopic organisation of the motor cortex in the precentral gyrus). Diagnosis is by lumbar puncture (to demonstrate a normal CSF opening pressure) followed by head computed tomography/magnetic resonance imaging (CT/MRI), showing enlarged ventricles. Treatment is with ventriculoperitoneal shunting.

28. Complications of blood transfusion

D. Stop the transfusion, take blood cultures and provide supportive measures

Immediate transfusion reactions can be severe and potentially fatal. There are several possibilities for acute fevers during a transfusion. Rarely this may indicate an acute transfusion reaction, potentially due to ABO compatibility, most commonly due to an error in administering the correct blood to the correct patient. This reaction will occur within the first few minutes of a transfusion and be characterised by shortness of breath, pain and a fever (but the patient in this scenario is on his second unit). Very rarely, a fever may be due to infection present in the blood product itself. A fever, especially following previous history of blood transfusion, may be due to a non-haemolytic transfusion reaction resulting from antibodies to the white blood cells.

In the acute setting initial management is vital to protect the patient. Initially this involves stopping the blood transfusion and providing supportive therapy to the patient in terms of oxygen, hydration and ventilatory support as necessary. Senior help should be sought immediately, and the laboratory contacted to trace the blood to patient stocks. Steroids and antihistamines may be useful in calming the immune response in the short term. All transfusion-related adverse events must be reported to a centralised database that aims to improve overall safety.

29. Diagnosis of numbness

C. Hypocalcaemia

Hypoparathyroidism is a relatively common, and transient, complication of subtotal thyroidectomy. Reduced levels of parathyroid hormone result in high phosphate levels and low calcium levels. The symptoms of hypocalcaemia include perioral paraesthesia, muscular cramping and depression.

Signs of hypocalcaemia include carpopedal spasm when a blood pressure cuff is inflated over the brachial artery (Trousseau's sign) and facial twitching when the facial nerve is excited by tapping above the parotid gland (Chvostek's sign). If the patient is stable and only suffering mild symptoms, the condition can be corrected using oral calcium supplementation. If the patient is very symptomatic, a 10-mL intravenous dose of 10% calcium gluconate can be administered. Approximately 1% of patients will develop permanent hypoparathyroidism following subtotal thyroidectomy.

The most common cause of hypocalcaemia is hypoalbuminaemia with a normal ionised calcium concentration (hence why it is important to correct calcium concentrations according to serum albumin). Other causes include alkalosis, vitamin D deficiency, chronic renal failure, pseudohypoparathyroidism, acute pancreatitis and hypomagnesaemia.

Pseudohypoparathyroidism is an autosomal dominant condition characterised by end-organ resistance to parathyroid hormone. Features include mental retardation, short stature and short fourth and fifth metacarpals, accompanied by a low parathyroid hormone (PTH), low calcium and high phosphate levels. Pseudopseudohypoparathyroidism describes the condition where you get all the phenotypic features of pseudohypoparathyroidism but in conjunction with a normal biochemistry.

30. Diagnosis of postural hypotension

D. Short Synacthen test

This patient presents with features suggestive of adrenocortical insufficiency, the diagnosis of which may be confirmed using the short Synacthen test.

31. Management of delirium

D. Reducing dose of chlordiazepoxide and intravenous Pabrinex

Delirium tremens is caused by sudden alcohol withdrawal and presents with agitation, confusion and hallucinations. Autonomic symptoms such as tachycardia, sweating and nausea commonly co-exist. Lilliputian hallucinations (seeing little people) are characteristic. (Named after the island of Lilliput in Jonathan Swift's novel *Gulliver's Travels*, where the inhabitants were "not 6 inches high".) If untreated, seizures can occur. Chlordiazepoxide (a benzodiazepine) treats the agitation and can prevent seizure occurrence, whilst vitamin B replacement aims to prevent Wernicke encephalopathy and the irreversible Korsakoff psychosis from developing (both caused by lack of vitamin B_1, levels of which can dramatically drop in alcohol withdrawal, especially with the likely malnourished state of the alcoholic). Pabrinex is not available orally, only intravenously.

Chlordiazepoxide is commonly given as a high dose initially and then tailed off over 4–5 days.

Delirium, from Latin *delirare* = to be crazy (from *de* = away from + *lira* = path)

32. Liver function tests

E. Prolonged prothrombin time

The synthetic function of the liver is assessed either by the clotting pathway, as vitamin K–dependent clotting factors are absorbed via the liver, or through serum albumin levels. If the liver is not functioning properly, clotting becomes deranged and the serum albumin concentrations decrease. Serum albumin, however, can act as an acute-phase protein and be reduced in many inflammatory or infective situations. Alanine transferase and alkaline phosphatase are markers of hepatocellular damage.

33. Diagnosis of cough

B. Bronchiectasis

Bronchiectasis is an abnormal permanent dilatation of bronchi secondary to destruction of the bronchial wall. It is usually an acquired condition as a consequence of recurrent and/or severe infections. It may result from an underlying genetic condition or congenital defect of airway defences. Patients present with a chronic cough that may be associated with large amounts of thick, yellow, foul-smelling sputum and sometimes haemoptysis. When there are large amounts of sputum in the bronchiectatic spaces, inspiratory squeaks and crackles and rhonchi are heard on chest auscultation.

34. Diagnosis of skin lesions

D. Skin scrapings to be sent for microscopy culture and sensitivities

This patient has tinea corporis in association with tinea pedis. Tinea is a fungal dermatophyte that can infect the skin in any area of the body. Common infections are tinea pedis (athlete's foot) and tinea cruris (fungal infection of the medial upper thighs). Tinea corporis is rarer and presents as a growing, flat, erythematous lesion with an inflamed scaly border. It usually spreads from tinea pedis on the same patient. Tinea pedis itself is usually transmitted by infected keratinous debris, e.g. from shower floors. Differentials of tinea corporis include granuloma annulare and erythema annulare. Fungal infection is confirmed by skin scrapings being examined under the microscope for fungal hyphae. Swabs are unlikely to pick up fungal material, and biopsies are excessive at this stage. If the skin scraping does not show a fungal element and the lesion does not respond to empirical antifungal therapy, a punch biopsy may elucidate the cause and nature of the lesion and direct further therapy.

Tinea, from Latin *tinea* = growing worm

35. Electrocardiogram

D. Inferior

Anterolateral infarcts typically show changes in V4–6, I and aVL. Anteroseptal infarcts show changes in V1–4. Anterior infarcts are shown in leads V1–6, I and aVL. Posterior infarcts rarely lead to substantial changes other than perhaps a raised R-wave in V1.

It helps to remember what the leads are measuring. II, III and aVF (F for feet) are measuring the downwards-pointing inferior myocardium. The chest leads and I measure the outwards pointing anterior myocardium (V1– 4 right, V4–6 and I left). Infarcts usually occur in the harder-working left ventricle, the right side of which is the interventricular septum.

36. Diagnosis of neurological dysfunction

D. Syringomyelia

Let's start with the easy ones to rule out. Viral transverse myelitis is an acute illness and would not develop so insidiously. Cervical spondylosis is predominantly a disease that affects those over 50, and the arm signs would be more of a "radiculopathic" nature – shooting pains or paraesthesia in a nerve root distribution. This leaves two illnesses commonly presenting in young females: psychogenic symptoms and multiple sclerosis (MS) and syringomyelia. Localising the potential lesion would identify the cervical spinal cord as the location (lower motor neurone signs in the arms, potentially upper motor neurone signs in the legs), so MS is a possibility. However, it does not sound like a normal relapse, as things have slowly progressed over 6 months with no clear resolution, and the symptoms and signs appear to be symmetrical. There is no evidence of brainstem, cerebellar or optic nerve involvement, and the white matter tracts appear to be less clearly involved than the lower motor neurones. Regarding the possibility of a psychogenic cause, the symptoms are not in a bizarre inexplicable distribution, and there are convincing examination signs, so that leaves syringomyelia.

In syringomyelia, the central canal of the spinal cord distends and begins to damage neurones by pressure effect. The syrinx (the swelling itself) starts in the cervical cord and can spread both superiorly and inferiorly. The first neurones to be damaged are the pain and temperature neurones bilaterally as their small axons cross the midline near the canal. As this only happens at the level of the syrinx and not above or below and light touch and proprioception are spared, this causes the classic pattern of cape-like dissociated sensory loss. The anterior horn cell neurones (i.e. lower motor neurones) can also become damaged, giving a lower motor neurone picture at the level of the syrinx (wasting, absent reflexes), then long tract signs may develop later as the syrinx grows (upper motor neurone signs in the legs). Syringomyelia is usually associated with either a history of trauma to the spine or Chiari malformation, in which the cerebellar tonsils (at the very least) lie below the level of the foramen magnum. In this patient, she may well have the malformation, which may also explain the occipital headaches.

Syringomyelia, from Latin *syrinx* = pipe or tube

Hans Chiari, Austrian pathologist (1851-1916)

37. Management of ischaemic stroke

E. Warfarin

Aspirin started immediately after an acute ischaemic stroke reduces early recurrence and has a small benefit on long-term outcome. Statin therapy has been shown to be beneficial even without high cholesterol prior to treatment. Warfarin is not indicated here, as there is no atrial fibrillation, it is her first stroke and there is nothing sinister in the past medical history suggesting a drastic predisposition to thrombus formation. (Furthermore, warfarin is only indicated if there is co-existing valve disease; in the absence of such pathology, a direct oral anticoagulant [DOAC] may be more appropriate.) Angiotensin-converting enzyme (ACE) inhibitor therapy has a beneficial effect even if the blood pressure was previously normal. The European Carotid Surgery Trial showed that carotid stenosis above 70% should be operated on by endarterectomy to deliver maximal benefit in prevention of further transient ischaemic attacks (TIAs) or strokes, outweighing the risks of surgery.

38. Malignant melanoma

D. Colour different from that of other moles on the patient

Many people like to remember the ABCDE rule when it comes to moles and melanoma: asymmetry, border irregularity, colour irregularity (*within the mole in question*), diameter > 7 mm and evolution of lesion (size, shape, colour). Patients will often have moles of several different shades, all of which are benign, and therefore this is not a concerning feature. As well as the ABCDE, other concerning features are inflammation or border erythema, bleeding or oozing, itching, elevation and altered sensation. Risk factors in the patients themselves include having multiple (>50) melanocytic naevi, dysplastic naevus syndrome, excessive sun exposure, positive past or family history and type I skin.

The skin types, as described by T.B. Fitzpatrick (current dermatologist, Harvard) in 1975, are:

Type I	White, very fair, freckles	Always burns, never tans
Type II	White, fair	Usually burns, tans with difficulty
Type III	Beige	Sometimes mild burn, gradually tans
Type IV	Beige with brown tint	Rarely burns, tans with ease
Type V	Dark brown	Very rarely burns, tans very easily
Type VI	Black	Never burns, tans very easily

39. Nipple discharge

E. Urgent computed tomography (CT) of the brain

The cardinal features of hyperprolactinaemia are galactorrhoea (milk discharge) and hypogonadism. Hyperprolactinaemia causes milk production, and patients present with a nipple discharge that is not associated with breastfeeding. Hypogonadism presents with secondary amenorrhoea and anovulation with infertility in women and decreased libido and lethargy in men. There are many causes of hyperprolactinaemia, and one of them is drug induced. Dopamine antagonists (e.g. antipsychotics, antidepressants, antiemetics) are known to increase prolactin concentrations. Breast examination should be performed to exclude breast malignancy. Primary hypothyroidism causes thyroid-releasing hormone (TRH)–induced prolactin excess, and thus a thyroid function test should be performed. A computed tomography (CT) scan of the hypothalamus and pituitary gland should be carried out only if serum prolactin is persistently high (1000 mU/L) to detect a prolactin-secreting pituitary tumour (prolactinoma).

The treatment of hyperprolactinaemia secondary to pituitary disease involves dopamine agonists (bromocriptine) followed by surgery to remove the tumour if indicated.

40. Palpitations

D. Thyroid function tests

Despite the lack of other signs of hyperthyroidism, thyroid function tests are an important part of the investigation. Hyperthyroidism results in a hyperdynamic circulation. This increases tissue oxygen consumption, causes peripheral vasodilatation and, in response, raises cardiac output. T_4 and T_3 also directly stimulate cardiac output. The resultant tachycardia, contractility and directly raised oxygen demand can strain a weakened heart. Palpitations, atrial fibrillation, shortness of breath (from left ventricular failure), aggravated angina, a pulmonary mid-diastolic "high-flow" murmur and cardiomegaly are the cardiac signs of hyperthyroidism.

Haematinics (iron, B$_{12}$, folate) will indicate anaemia due to impaired erythropoiesis and could be requested, as anaemia can cause these symptoms.

There is no indication for a troponin, as the symptoms are painless and not acute.

Palpitations, from Latin *palpitatio* = throbbing

41. Diagnosis of endocrine disease

A. Growth hormone levels during an oral glucose tolerance test

This patient has acromegaly. Features of acromegaly include swelling of the hands and feet, lower jaw protrusion, macroglossia (large tongue), bitemporal hemianopia, carpal tunnel syndrome, hypertension, hyperglycaemia and cardiomegaly.

In health, high plasma glucose levels feed back to suppress growth hormone (GH) secretion. In acromegaly, there is autonomous secretion of GH, usually from a pituitary adenoma that escapes the control of negative feedback. The definitive test for diagnosis is GH levels during an oral glucose tolerance test (typically a full pituitary blood panel, including insulin-like growth factor-1 [IGF-1] is undertaken at first presentation). Blood samples for GH are taken at a fixed interval after ingestion of the glucose. GH is inhibited by a rise in glucose, and thus GH should be undetectable. In acromegaly, however, GH secretion is not suppressed and the level remains high. The failure to suppress GH levels to below 1 μg/L 2 hours after a 75-g oral glucose bolus is considered a positive result. Random GH levels are not helpful in the diagnosis, as it is secreted in a markedly pulsatile manner, and it is affected by stress, sleep, puberty and pregnancy. Magnetic resonance imaging (MRI) scanning of the pituitary fossa is useful, as hypersecretion of GH is normally from a pituitary tumour. Panhypopituitarism may also be caused by a pituitary tumour. IGF-1 concentration is high with excessive GH secretion, but in 25% of the cases, IGF-1 remains normal with increased GH secretion.

Acromegaly, from Greek *acro* = extremities + *megalos* = large

42. Emollient use

A. Acne vulgaris

Emollients, ranging from the thin aqueous cream to the far thicker "50:50" (white soft paraffin and liquid paraffin in 50% proportions), are useful in conditions featuring dry or scaly skin. They rehydrate the skin, reinstitute the surface lipid layer and should be taken seriously as part of the management of dry or scaling conditions, without which other topical or systemic treatments would be less effective. Patient preference is a big factor, and there is a wide range on the market; therefore patients should be offered many to find which ones suit them. Contact dermatitis, eczema and psoriasis would all generally benefit from use of emollients by virtue of featuring dryness as part of the rashes. Emollients can also be applied to wounds during the healing process, and this is encouraged by some surgeons. Acne vulgaris, however, is related to increased sebum production, which can block pores of sebaceous glands and become infected and inflamed. Therefore, emollients are only likely to make matters worse.

Emollient, from Latin *emollire* = to soften

43. Medications in acute renal failure

A. Amlodipine

Diclofenac is a non-steroidal anti-inflammatory drug (NSAID), which can be nephrotoxic by interfering with renal blood supply at the efferent arteriole, an effect magnified in hypovolaemia. Digoxin is excreted by the kidney and thus can have increased toxicity in renal impairment – hence the dose may need to be lowered. Furosemide is a potent diuretic and is likely to increase hypovolaemia and therefore should be stopped in this instance. Metformin can induce a metabolic acidosis and so should be stopped if the creatinine level is above 150. Amlodipine is a calcium channel blocker, a relatively safe family of anti-hypertensives that does not need to be altered in renal failure, whereas angiotensin-converting enzyme (ACE) inhibitors, beta-blockers and thiazide diuretics should all be used carefully in acute renal failure. If the patient becomes hypotensive, however, then it should be considered whether to stop the amlodipine for that reason.

44. Rectal bleeding

C. Anal fissure

Anal fissures can occur in isolation, often following a period of constipation, or on a background of inflammatory bowel disease (such as Crohn's disease and ulcerative colitis). It is most common in young people aged 20–30 and presents as an intense pain on defecation that may last for up to 1 hour afterwards. The pain is caused by a tear in the mucosa and muscle spasm during the passage of stools. Treatment is initially with stool softeners to attempt to allow the mucosa to heal naturally. Glyceryl trinitrite (GTN) topically may provide relief of symptoms, and botulinum toxin can be used where GTN fails.

45. Signs of liver disease

C. Kayser–Fleischer rings

Kayser–Fleischer rings are seen in Wilson's disease, in which copper is deposited in vital organs due to an error in metabolism, which means that it cannot be secreted into the bile. Kayser–Fleischer rings are due to the deposition of copper in Descemet's membrane, which is located between the corneal stroma and endothelium in the eye. They appear as brown-green rings around the iris and are seen in up to 90% of patients with Wilson's disease. In most patients they can only be seen using a slit lamp examination, although they may be visible with the naked eye in patients with light blue eyes and in patients with advanced disease.

46. Indications for haemodialysis in acute renal failure

B. Hypertension > 220 mmHg systolic or 160 mmHg diastolic

Hypertension is not acutely life threatening, whereas acidosis, refractory hyperkalaemia, pulmonary oedema and uraemic pericarditis can potentially be life-threatening. Reliable pharmacological therapies that are not overcome by the ongoing renal failure exist for hypertension, whereas they do not for severe acidosis, persistent hyperkalaemia, refractory pulmonary oedema or uraemic pericarditis. Vasodilation and decreasing vascular resistance are not impossible in renal failure. Acidosis can be temporarily ameliorated by use of sodium bicarbonate, but it is unclear whether this helps in the long run, especially if the renal failure does not reverse. Severe hyperkalaemia can lead to ventricular fibrillation and result in cardiac arrest – hence monitoring should be instituted, calcium gluconate given to stabilise the cardiac membrane and insulin with dextrose and calcium resonium given to lower serum potassium. However, if the renal failure does not reverse, the potassium will continue to rise. Morphine can relieve respiratory distress, and nitrates can vasodilate and pool blood away from the lungs in pulmonary oedema, but if the renal failure does not reverse, dialysis will be needed to remove the excess fluid. Acute rises in urea can lead to pericarditis and even pericardial effusions and tamponade, and only haemofiltration or haemodialysis can reduce the serum urea to prevent this if the kidneys do not soon recover.

47. Sexually transmitted infections

A. Bacterial vaginosis (BV)

BV is not a sexually transmitted infection, but rather an imbalance of the polymicrobial vaginal flora. There is often a preponderance of mixed anaerobic flora (e.g. *Gardnerella vaginalis* and *Mycoplasma hominis*). It is often asymptomatic but can cause a creamy-grey discharge with a fishy odour. There is no itching. The diagnosis of BV is by the Amsel criteria (at least three of the following): homogenous discharge, clue cells on microscopy, pH of vaginal fluid >4.5 and release of a fishy odour on addition of 10% potassium hydroxide to the discharge. Clue cells are epithelial cells with bacteria adherent to the surface. BV can be treated with antibiotics (e.g. metronidazole), but there is a high rate of recurrence.

48. Systemic lupus erythematosus

E. Red rash across the cheeks that is worse in summer

Anterior uveitis often affects patients with ankylosing spondylitis or other HLA-B27–associated arthropathies. Anti-ribonucleoprotein antibodies can be involved in systemic lupus erythematosus (SLE) but are more suggestive of the diagnosis of mixed connective tissue disease, which can give features of scleroderma, myositis and lupus. The arthropathy of SLE is normally non-erosive, and erosions are more suggestive of rheumatoid arthritis. Painful, palpable, purple lumps on the shins describes erythema nodosum, which may stand alone or be a feature of sarcoidosis or inflammatory bowel disease or follow various infective diseases, e.g. post-streptococcal.

The red rash across the cheeks, which spares the nasolabial folds, describes the classic malar, or "butterfly", rash of SLE. Importantly, to make a diagnosis of SLE, the American College of Rheumatology criteria are used, which require 4 of 11 criteria to be fulfilled either serially or simultaneously (remembered by "A RASH POINts MD"):

- **A**rthralgia
- **R**enal disease → Nephrotic syndrome
- **A**ntinuclear antibody
- **S**erositis → Pleurisy, pleural effusion, pericarditis
- **H**aematology disorders → Pancytopenia
- **P**hotosensitivity
- **O**ral ulcers
- **I**mmunology (autoantibodies) → Anti-dsDNA, anti-Smith
- **N**eurological problems → Depression, psychosis
- **M**alar rash
- **D**iscoid rash

49. Uraemia

D. Spider naevi

Severe chronic uraemia can lead to a subtle pale-yellow shade of skin that is described as "lemon yellow" (due to the combination of anaemia and urochrome deposition) or sometimes "uraemic frost" (due to the deposition of urea crystals in the skin). Uraemic encephalopathy can cause a clouding of consciousness and an acute confusional state, as well as myoclonic jerks, and this can progress to seizures and coma if not reversed. Hiccoughing (persistent hiccups) is also seen. Spider naevi are seen in chronic liver disease and are not a feature of uraemia.

B. AVP deficiency (cranial diabetes insipidus)

Antidiuretic hormone (ADH) is secreted from the posterior pituitary gland in response to a high plasma osmolality, hypovolaemia or stress. Its main function is to stimulate the reabsorption of water from the collecting ducts of the nephron into the circulation. This results in a reduction in plasma osmolality and urine output and an increase in urine osmolality and blood pressure. Diabetes insipidus (DI) is a condition caused by either an absolute lack of ADH secretion (cranial DI) or renal insensitivity to its actions (nephrogenic DI). DI usually presents with massive polyuria, as water cannot be reabsorbed from the collecting ducts. As a result, patients with diabetes insipidus are often dehydrated and consume massive amounts of water in order to maintain their fluid balance. Other conditions that may present in a similar manner include diabetes mellitus, hypercalcaemia and psychogenic polydipsia. DI is suggested by a plasma osmolality >300 mOsm/kg with a urine osmolality <600 mOsm/kg. DI is usually diagnosed using the water deprivation test. This involves measuring the patient's urine volume, concentration and plasma osmolality whilst depriving the patient of water. A positive result is recorded when water deprivation fails to increase the concentration of urine due to a lack of ADH or insensitivity to its actions. If the initial test is positive, the patient is given a dose of desmopressin – a synthetic ADH analogue. If the patient concentrates their urine in response to desmopressin, the defect must be central, and a diagnosis of cranial DI can be made. If, however, the urine is not concentrated following desmopressin administration, there is end-organ resistance to ADH, i.e. nephrogenic DI.

Diabetes insipidus, from Greek *diabainein* = to siphon + Latin *in* = not + *sapere* = to taste

In other words, to pass tasteless urine

Practice paper 5: Questions

1. Alzheimer's disease

Which of the following statements regarding Alzheimer's disease is FALSE?

A Cholinesterase inhibitor may halt progression
B Computed tomography (CT) or magnetic resonance imaging (MRI) may show medial temporal atrophy
C Pathologically, extracellular beta-amyloid plaques are seen
D Pathologically, intracellular tau-protein neurofibrillary tangles are seen
E Short-term memory impairment is an early symptom

2. Antibiotics with warfarin

A 78-year-old man taking warfarin for a metallic aortic valve presents with 5 days of cough productive of purulent sputum, fever, anorexia and confusion. He is diagnosed with community-acquired pneumonia and is admitted for antibiotic therapy.

Which of the following antibiotics does NOT interact with warfarin?

A Ciprofloxacin
B Clarithromycin
C Gentamicin
D Metronidazole
E Rifampicin

3. Management of hyperglycaemia

A 32-year-old man with known type 1 diabetes mellitus presents to the emergency department with nausea and vomiting. His blood glucose level was 24 mmol/L, with high blood ketones and K^+ 4.5 mmol/L.

Which of the following management options is NOT appropriate in this patient on the first day?

A Commence intravenous 0.9% normal saline of 1 L bolus
B Start intravenous insulin infusion at a rate of 1 U/kg/hour
C Start intravenous K^+ supplement 40 mmol/L to maintain K at 3.5–5.5
D Monitor blood glucose hourly
E Consider urinary catheter

DOI: 10.1201/9781003648222-9

4. Burns management

You are working on the burns unit, and a patient requires a split-thickness skin graft to cover a defect on the dorsum of the left hand secondary to a full-thickness scald burn 7 days ago. TBSA 0.5%. The wound looks erythematous and sloughy and feels warm to touch. Which part of skin graft take will infection disrupt?

A Adhesion
B Plasmic imbibition
C Re-vascularisation

D Neovascularisation
E Remodelling

5. Investigation of hypothyroidism

A 43-year-old woman presents to her GP with a 3-month history of lethargy and low mood. She noticed that she had gained 2 stones over the past 2 months, despite having a normal appetite. On examination, she looked pale with periorbital puffiness, with a bitemporal hemianopia. Her thyroid gland was not palpable. Her thyroid function tests showed TSH 0.3 (range 0.5–5.5) mU/L, T_4 3 (range 4.5–12.5) µg/dL.

Which investigation would be most useful in the diagnosis?

A 99m technetium (^{99m}Tc) scintigraphy scans
B Magnetic resonance imaging (MRI) of the brain
C Thyroid peroxidase antibodies
D Thyroid-stimulating hormone (TSH) receptor-blocking antibodies
E Ultrasound of the thyroid gland

6. Sickle cell disease

A 16-year-old boy with known sickle cell disease presents with painful hands bilaterally after being out early in the morning for a run. He is otherwise systemically well.

What should be your immediate management?

A Joint aspiration
B Malaria screen
C Referral to rheumatology

D Rehydration and analgesia
E X-rays

7. Skin cancer

Which of the following is FALSE about basal cell carcinomas?

A They typically present as a nodule with rounded edges and telangiectasia
B They readily metastasise to bone
C They are the most common skin cancer variant
D Lesions <2 cm in diameter are excised with a 4-mm margin
E Gorlin syndrome is typically linked with multiple BCCs

8. Skin manifestations of systemic disease

A 16-year-old girl presents to the GP with an itchy rash. This is located on both forearms, and examination reveals evidence of blistering. She has a history of coeliac disease but is otherwise systemically well.

What is the most likely diagnosis?

A Acrodermatitis enteropathica
B Candidiasis
C Dermatitis herpetiformis
D Leucoplakia
E Linea nigra

9. Hepatic haemangioma

A 32-year-old woman undergoes a contrast-enhanced CT scan of her abdomen to look for a cause of lower abdominal pain. Although no obvious cause of the pain is found, there is a small, cavernous haemangioma of the liver.

What is the next step in management of this lesion?

A Anticoagulation with lifelong aspirin
B Chemotherapy
C Head CT to rule out cerebral haemangiomas
D No treatment necessary
E Surgical resection

10. Oxygen therapy

A 65-year-old man with a long-standing history of chronic obstructive pulmonary disease was admitted to the hospital with an acute exacerbation. His observations include temperature 37.5°C, pulse rate 120 bpm, blood pressure 140/90 mmHg, respiratory rate 28/min and saturations 84% on room air. An arterial blood gas shows pH 7.31, PaO_2 4.6 kPa, $PaCO_2$ 8.3 kPa and bicarbonate 25.2 mmol/L.

What is the most appropriate percentage of O_2 to be given initially?

A 28%
B 35%
C 40%
D 60%
E 100%

11. Polycystic kidney disease

A 43-year-old man has just been diagnosed with polycystic kidney disease and is keen to know about potential risks or associated health problems.

Which of the following is NOT an extra-renal complication of polycystic kidney disease?

A Bladder diverticuli
B Cerebral aneurysms
C Hepatic cysts
D Mitral valve prolapse
E Pancreatic cysts

12. Hip pain

A 28-year-old woman has recently started exercising more frequently at the gym. She has not noticed any injuries. She has attended the GP practice, as over the last couple of days she's had increasing pain in her left hip, and now has an antalgic gait throughout the day only relieved with rest. She is well otherwise. On examination there is no discernible signs to see other than pain placing axial pressure on the hip.

What is the most likely diagnosis?

A Septic arthritis
B Osteoarthritis
C Rheumatoid arthritis
D Osteosarcoma
E Iliotibial band syndrome

13. Hyperbilirubinaemia

During a routine medical for a work placement, a GP discovered that a 33-year-old man who was otherwise fit and healthy had a raised bilirubin level. He otherwise had entirely normal liver function tests and a full blood count. He had no history of foreign travel or drug or alcohol abuse. Repeated blood tests 1 month later showed a similar picture.

What is the most likely diagnosis?

A Crigler–Najjar syndrome
B Gilbert's disease
C Haemolytic anaemia
D Hepatitis B
E Pancreatic cancer

14. Drugs used in cardiac arrest

Which of the following drugs is used during cardiac arrest to improve the coronary perfusion pressure?

A Adrenaline
B Amiodarone
C Atropine
D Calcium gluconate
E Magnesium sulphate

15. Management of thyrotoxicosis

A 35-year-old woman presents to the GP with increased weight loss over the past 2 months, with lid retraction, exophthalmos and double vision. Her T_3 and T_4 are raised.

Which of the following is the first-line treatment in this patient?

A Beta-blockers
B Carbimazole therapy
C Intravenous hydrocortisone
D Radioactive iodine therapy
E Subtotal thyroidectomy

16. Haemoptysis

A 26-year-old woman from sub-Saharan Africa presents with 2 months of haemoptysis and lethargy. In the last month she has lost half a stone in weight, and she complains that she frequently soaks the bedsheets with sweat. She has a negligible smoking history.

What is the most likely diagnosis?

A Lung cancer
B Lymphoma
C *Pneumocystis* pneumonia
D Pulmonary embolism
E Tuberculosis

17. Arterial blood gases

A 33-year-old man presents to the emergency department with acute shortness of breath. He appears exhausted and unable to provide a clear history. An arterial blood gas reading shows pH 7.33, PaO_2 7.3 kPa, $PaCO_2$ 6.9 kPa and bicarbonate 26 mmol/L on room air (reference range: pH 7.35–7.45, PaO_2 11–13 kPa, $PaCO_2$ 4.7-6.0 kPa, HCO_3^- 22–26 mEq/L).

What abnormality do these results represent?

A Metabolic acidosis
B Metabolic alkalosis
C Respiratory acidosis
D Respiratory alkalosis
E Type 1 respiratory failure

18. Dry eyes

A 38-year-old woman with a history of autoimmune thyroid disease presents with persistently dry eyes for over a year. She denies any arthralgia, rash, fatigue or any other symptoms. Schirmer's test reveals <10 mm wetting of filter paper in 5 minutes. Antibodies reveal positive antinuclear antibodies, with positive anti-Ro and anti-La antibodies.

Which of the following represents the best course of management?

A Artificial tears
B Hydroxychloroquine
C Steroids
D Surveillance
E Tear duct surgery

19. Management of shortness of breath

A 21-year-old woman is admitted to the emergency department with increasing shortness of breath after taking oral amoxicillin, which was started by her GP this morning for a chest infection. Chest auscultation reveals widespread wheeze bilaterally. Vascular access is secured.

Which of the following management options is NOT appropriate?

A Discontinue administration of the suspected drug
B Give intramuscular adrenaline immediately
C Give intravenous 5% dextrose immediately
D Give intravenous chlorphenamine
E Give intravenous hydrocortisone

20. Shoulder injury

A 29-year-old man has been preparing for his skiing holiday by practicing at a nearby dry ski slope. He has fallen on an outstretched right hand and immediately suffered pain in his right shoulder. It was a closed injury, but there was a prominent bulge to the anterior shoulder. He struggled to abduct his shoulder on examination and had loss of sensation at the lateral aspect of his shoulder.

What nerve is most likely injured?

A Median
B Axillary
C Radial
D Ulnar
E Musculocutaneous

21. Haemophilia

Which clotting factor is deficient in haemophilia A?

A VII
B VIII
C IX

D XI
E vWF

22. Gastrointestinal pathology

A histology report for a specimen taken from the colon of a 24-year-old woman states "patchy areas of transmural non-caseating granulomatous inflammation".

What disease process does this suggest?

A Colonic adenocarcinoma
B Crohn's disease
C Irritable bowel syndrome

D Tuberculosis
E Ulcerative colitis

23. Blood film

Which of the following conditions do NOT cause a leucoerythroblastic picture on blood film?

A Chronic myeloid leukaemia
B Megaloblastic anaemia
C Metastatic spread to the bone marrow
D Myeloma
E Tuberculosis

24. Lung cancer

A 55-year-old woman presents to the emergency department with a 1-month history of shortness of breath and weakness in both lower limbs. She has a 15-pack/year smoking history and was recently diagnosed with diabetes by her GP. She has no other significant past medical history. On examination, there is reduced air entry on the left lower lung zone. Her chest X-ray shows a mass lesion on the left lower lobe.

An arterial blood gas reading shows pH 7.53, PaO_2 8.6 kPa, $PaCO_2$ 5.3 kPa, bicarbonate 30.2 mmol/L (reference range: pH 7.35–7.45, PaO_2 11–13 kPa, $PaCO_2$ 4.7–6.0 kPa, HCO_3^- 22–26 mEq/L).

The blood result shows Na^+ 137 mmol/L, K^+ 2.3, urea 4.8 mmol/L, creatinine 108 μmol/L.

A CT of the chest reveals a tumour invading the left lung, and a percutaneous lung biopsy confirms the diagnosis of lung cancer.

What biochemical abnormalities are shown, and what is the most likely histology of the lung cancer?

A Metabolic acidosis, non–small cell carcinoma
B Metabolic alkalosis, small cell carcinoma
C Metabolic alkalosis, non–small cell carcinoma
D Respiratory alkalosis, small cell carcinoma
E Respiratory alkalosis, non–small cell carcinoma

25. Cavernous sinus lesions

Which of the following cranial nerves would be affected by pathology in the cavernous sinus?

A II, III, IV and VI
B III and V
C III, IV and VI
D III, IV, VI and ophthalmic and maxillary division of V
E III, IV, VI and V

26. Cognitive impairment

A 75-year-old man presents with a history of episodes of cognitive impairment and memory deficits. His daughter seems perplexed that at some times he seems entirely normal; however, some days he seems muddled and can't remember anything. He occasionally claims to see faces where there are none. He is a smoker and has COPD, but there is nothing else in his past medical history. On examination he has a slow tremor present in his left thumb when relaxed or distracted, but this is not present when he moves his arm. The arms appear to have a rigid tone, more on the left than on the right. The rest of the neurological and general examination appears normal.

Which of the following is the most likely cause?

A Depressive pseudodementia
B Frontotemporal dementia
C Korsakoff psychosis
D Lewy body dementia
E Vascular dementia

27. Complications of bone marrow transplant

One year after bone marrow transplantation from a matched donor to treat non-Hodgkin's lymphoma, a patient re-presents complaining of widespread skin irritation. The skin is exfoliated in areas and there is a maculopapular rash, while the fingers are becoming sclerotic. He has not been feeling himself for a while with episodes of diarrhoea and recurrent chest infections.

What is the most likely reason for this?

A Acute graft rejection
B Chronic graft-versus-host disease
C Herpes zoster infection
D New-onset scleroderma
E Side effect of immunosuppressants

28. Diagnosis of abdominal pain

A 24-year-old woman presents with a 3-month history of vague right upper quadrant pains. She has also noticed an abnormal vaginal discharge since starting a new sexual relationship 4 months ago. On examination there is a hepatic friction rub.

What is the most likely diagnosis?

A Fitz-Hugh–Curtis syndrome
B Hepatitis C
C HIV
D Liver abscess
E Liver infarct

29. Diagnosis of cough

A 36-year-old man has a 1-month history of a non-productive dry cough. He also reports increasing dyspnoea on exertion for the past 2 weeks. He was a known intravenous drug user. Chest auscultation is unremarkable. He is referred to the medical assessment unit for a chest X-ray, which shows bilateral symmetrical interstitial infiltrates. A subsequent HIV test is positive.

Which of the following is the most likely causative agent?

A *Aspergillus fumigates*
B Cytomegalovirus
C *Histoplasma capsulatum*
D *Pneumocystis jirovecii*
E *Staphylococcus aureus*

30. Palpitations

A 28-year-old woman with known neurofibromatosis type I presents to her GP with palpitations and recurrent headaches that are not relieved by paracetamol. She also feels dizzy and becomes sweaty during these episodes. Her blood pressure is found to be 220/120 mmHg.

What is the most likely diagnosis?

A Acromegaly   D Thyrotoxicosis
B Carcinoid syndrome   E Phaeochromocytoma
C Cushing's disease

31. Diagnosis of neurological dysfunction

A 28-year-old Afro-Caribbean pregnant woman presents with a 2-month history of tingling in her feet and difficulty walking, which has progressed so that she is barely able to walk. She came to Britain 3 years ago from West Africa and has struggled to find work since arriving. She is 5 months pregnant, has a 2-year-old son and lives in a flat with her boyfriend. She has no significant past medical history other than various diarrhoeal illnesses when living in Africa. On examination, she looks thin and the conjunctiva are pale. There are no cranial nerve abnormalities or abnormalities on the arms. In the legs, there is an increase in tone in the legs, with a marked weakness to about grade 3 or 4 throughout both legs, which is worse in the ankles. Knee jerks appear brisk, although the ankle jerks are hard to elicit and appear absent. Plantar reflexes are upgoing. There is a loss of light touch to just above the ankles, and there is absent proprioception and vibration sense in the big toe joints.

Which of the following is the most likely diagnosis?

A Diabetic polyneuropathy
B Guillain–Barré syndrome
C HIV-related polyneuropathy
D Subacute combined degeneration of the cord
E Tabes dorsalis

32. Diagnosis of skin lesions

A 60-year-old man presents with a 1.5-cm raised, pigmented lesion on his right arm. He is unsure how long it has been there.

Which feature on dermoscopy would suggest a malignant melanoma rather than a benign naevus or a pigmented seborrhoeic keratosis?

A Erythema of border
B Granular surface
C Irregular pigment network
D Stuck-on appearance
E Telangiectasia

33. Malignant melanoma

A 60-year-old Caucasian woman who recently moved from Zimbabwe presents with a growing pigmented lesion about 1 cm across with an irregular border and a raised, darker patch within. You suspect melanoma and excise the lesion.

Which of the following features of the tumour is the most informative prognosis indicator?

A Colour
B Diameter
C Asymmetry

D Invasive depth
E Bleeding

34. Electrocardiogram

Whilst on call, you are asked to review an ECG. It shows a long QT interval followed by a burst of QRS complexes at 300 bpm with an overlying waxing and waning R-wave amplitude, after which the ECG reverts back to its previous pattern. The patient feels well, and observations are stable.

You conclude that this was an episode of torsade de pointes. Which of the following would you not consider doing?

A Advise the nurses to perform hourly observations
B Check the drug chart for possible causes
C Provide immediate direct cardioversion
D Discuss with cardiology
E Transfer to cardiac monitor bed

35. Diagnosis of chest infection

A 75-year-old man presents with a 5-day history of cough productive of green sputum, mild right-sided chest pain, worsening breathlessness and, in the last day or so, confusion. He is previously fit and well with no background of dementia. He was in hospital 2 months ago for an elective hernia repair. On examination he has coarse crepitations at the right lung base, he has a respiratory rate of 34/min, a temperature of 38°C and an abbreviated mental test score of 6/10. Chest X-ray shows right lower zone consolidation and a small degree of blunting of the right costophrenic angle.

Which of the following is the likely diagnosis?

A Aspiration pneumonia
B Empyema
C Hospital-acquired pneumonia
D Mild or moderate community-acquired pneumonia
E Severe community-acquired pneumonia

36. Emergency management

A 16-year-old girl is seen by her general practitioner. She is lethargic and "not feeling her usual self" according to her parents. On examination, she has a stiff neck and a non-blanching purpuric rash on her trunk and legs.

Which of the following is the best course of action?

A Expectant management until there is deterioration
B Intramuscular benzylpenicillin and call ambulance
C Intramuscular benzylpenicillin and review in 12 hours
D Intravenous lorazepam and call ambulance
E Oral penicillin and review in 24 hours

37. Investigation of shortness of breath

A 53-year-old retired truck driver presents to the general practitioner with a 3-month history of productive cough. He also complains of gradual onset of shortness of breath on exertion. He has to stop for breath after walking about 100 metres on level ground. He is a heavy smoker but is otherwise fit and well.

Which of the following investigations would be most useful in establishing the cause of his symptoms?

A Chest X-ray   D Spirometry
B Electrocardiogram   E Sputum cytology
C Peak flow meter

38. Diagnosis of chest pain

A 54-year-old woman complains to her GP of repeated incidents of burning central chest pain, which mainly occurs when she lies down in bed at night. She is overweight with a body mass index of 40. She uses GTN occasionally, but it doesn't always relieve her symptoms. She doesn't report any shortness of breath or palpitations, and examination is unremarkable.

What is the most likely diagnosis?

A Angina   D Pancreatitis
B Gastro-oesophageal reflux disease   E Sleep apnoea
C Myocardial infarction

39. Hypoxia

You are called to see a 92-year-old woman on the ward. The patient is recovering from an exacerbation of heart failure. On arrival, the patient is on 15 L/min oxygen and an intravenous drip. You find the patient's oxygen saturation is reading 88% on pulse oximetry. She is having prolonged bouts of coughing, and the nurse looking after her reports that she seems physically weak and is delirious.

Which of the following would be the most appropriate initial course of action following your initial assessment?

A Check her fluid balance chart
B Start DNACPR discussions
C Keep checking the pulse oximeter hourly for deterioration
D Request a computed tomography (CT) pulmonary angiography
E Start her on antibiotics for hospital-acquired pneumonia

40. Management of hypothermia

A 46-year-old woman presents to the emergency department in a reduced state of consciousness. Her blood glucose level was 9 mmol/L. On examination, her body temperature was 33°C. She has non-pitting oedema on the skin of her hands, feet and eyelids. No obvious head injury is noticed. She has a thyroidectomy scar on her neck. She is bradycardic and hypotensive.

Bearing in mind the likely diagnosis, which of these is NOT appropriate in the initial management?

A High-flow oxygen if the patient is cyanosed
B Intravenous hydrocortisone
C Intravenous lorazepam
D Parenteral triiodothyronine, given slowly
E Warm blanket

41. Diagnosis of diabetes

A 45-year-old man presents to his GP with lethargy and polyuria for the past month. He has a strong family history of diabetes mellitus. A provisional diagnosis of diabetes mellitus is made.

Which of the following investigations is NOT useful in establishing the diagnosis?

A Fasting glucose level
B HbA1C level
C Oral glucose tolerance test
D Random glucose level
E Urine ketones

42. Medication review

An obese 58-year-old woman presented with fatigue and shortness of breath. She has recently been started on treatment for anxiety and has a background of asthma. Her oxygen saturation is 91% on air, and she is wheezy bilaterally. Which medication is most likely to be at fault?

A Citalopram
B Duloxetine
C Amitriptyline
D Propranolol
E Diazepam

43. Side effects of methotrexate

A 32-year-old woman is started on methotrexate for her newly diagnosed rheumatoid arthritis.

Which of the following is NOT true regarding side effects and contraindications of methotrexate?

A A baseline chest X-ray should be taken, as pulmonary fibrosis is a potential side effect
B Alcohol should be absolutely avoided whilst taking methotrexate
C Full blood count should be monitored, as neutropenia and myelosuppression are potential side effects
D Liver function tests should be monitored to watch for hepatic fibrosis
E Pregnancy should be avoided, and if considering having a baby, methotrexate should be switched to an alternative disease-modifying antirheumatic drug

44. Raised intracranial pressure

A 55-year-old man presents to the hospital with a 4-month history of headaches, which usually occur in the mornings. These are becoming more frequent and severe.

Which of the following would suggest increased intracranial pressure?

A Jaw claudication
B Kernig's sign
C Low opening pressure on lumbar puncture
D Relief of symptoms when lying down
E Transient bilateral visual loss

45. Bronchial carcinoma

A 53-year-old man is seen in the medical assessment unit with lethargy, nausea, polyuria and polydipsia. He's lost 2 stones over the period of 1 month and smokes 40 cigarettes per day. A chest X-ray shows a lung mass in the right lower lobe. His blood tests show a corrected calcium level of 3.1 mmol/L. Other causes of hypercalcaemia were excluded.

Which of the following cell types of bronchial carcinoma is most likely in this case?

A Adenocarcinoma
B Sarcomatoid carcinoma
C Small cell carcinoma
D Squamous cell carcinoma
E Large cell carcinoma

46. Neurological dysfunction

A 44-year-old woman who works in an office presents with a 2-month history of pains in her right hand and thumb weakness. The pains would shoot into her first three fingers, and initially she thought she was using bad typing technique; however, the pains progressed despite ergonomic keyboards and then she became weak in her thumb. She also says her first three fingers feel numb. On examination there is wasting of the thenar eminence, weakness of thumb abduction and reduced sensation in the thumb, index and middle finger and the lateral half of her fourth finger.

Which nerve or nerve root is affected?

A C6
B C8
C Median nerve
D Radial nerve
E Ulnar nerve

47. Diagnosis of rheumatoid arthritis

A 55-year-old woman presents to clinic with joint pain. She is concerned that it might be rheumatoid arthritis.

Which of the following clinical features is NOT used in the American College of Rheumatology criteria to diagnose rheumatoid arthritis and differentiate it from other causes of arthritis?

A Morning stiffness for 1 or more hours for more than 6 weeks
B Simultaneous symmetrical joint swelling for more than 6 weeks
C Three or more joints affected for more than 6 weeks
D Two hand joints (either metacarpophalangeal [MCP] or proximal inter-phalangeal [PIP]) involved for more than 6 weeks
E Ulnar deviation of one or more fingers for more than 6 weeks

48. Statistics

A new tumour marker is being tested for use in cholangiocarcinomas. In a trial, 40 patients have been tested. The trial produces 10 positive results and 30 negative results. Of the 10 positive results, 5 of them are false positives. Of the 30 negative results, 5 of them are false negatives.

What is the specificity of this test?

A 17%
B 50%
C 70%
D 83%
E 100%

49. Sepsis syndromes

A 43-year-old woman presents with a 1-week history of loin pain, suprapubic pain and dysuria. On examination she looks unwell and has a pulse of 110 bpm, blood pressure of 90/70 mmHg, respiratory rate of 24/min and temperature of 38.5°C. Bloods are taken for routine tests and blood cultures, a catheter passed and IV fluids and empirical antibiotics started. Later that day, blood cultures come back showing a Gram-negative rod. You note that in the last 3 hours she has only passed 30 mL of urine, and she is starting to show signs of confusion. Observations remain as they were earlier.

Which of the following terms best describes the patient's physiological status?

A Sepsis
B Septic shock
C Septicaemia
D Severe sepsis
E Systemic inflammatory response syndrome

50. Nephrotic syndrome

A 38-year-old man presents with fatigue, swelling of the eyelids and legs and frothy urine. His bloods appear normal except for an albumin level of 26 g/L (his albumin was normal on blood tests taken 1 year ago). You suspect nephrotic syndrome.

How would you confirm the diagnosis?

A Proteinuria on urine dipstick
B >1 g of protein lost in the urine over 24 hours
C >1 g of protein lost in the urine over 72 hours
D >3.5 g of protein lost in the urine over 24 hours
E >3.5 g of protein lost in the urine over 72 hours

Practice paper 5: Answers

1. Alzheimer's disease

A. Cholinesterase inhibitor may halt progression

Alzheimer's disease affects 5% of the population over 65 and is more common in females, Caucasians, those with positive family history or those with a degree of head trauma. Recent evidence has also linked poor sleep to the disease. Short-term memory impairment is indeed an early symptom of Alzheimer's disease. The medial temporal lobe includes the hippocampus and other limbic system areas, and degeneration of these areas contributes to the impairment of memory function. CT or single-photon emission CT (SPECT) or MRI may highlight such pathology. On microscopic pathological examination of the brain, both extracellular beta-amyloid plaques and tau-protein–based neurofibrillary tangles are seen. Degeneration of the basal forebrain nuclei also occurs in Alzheimer's disease, and cholinesterase inhibitors increase functional acetylcholine at synapses, thus temporarily improving memory dysfunction, especially in early disease. Cholinesterase inhibitors, however, do little to halt the progression of the underlying neuronal loss and thus progression of disease.

Alois Alzheimer, German psychiatrist (1864-1915)

2. Antibiotics with warfarin

C. Gentamicin

Quinolones such as ciprofloxacin, macrolides such as clarithromycin and the antibiotic metronidazole (used against anaerobic organisms) are all inhibitors of the cytochrome p450 metabolism system in the liver. They therefore inhibit hepatic metabolism of warfarin, leading to increased anticoagulant action and a raised international normalised ratio (INR). Other p450 inhibitors include omeprazole, sodium valproate and acute alcohol intake. Rifampicin is a cytochrome p450 inducer and so will enhance metabolism of warfarin and decrease the anticoagulant action. Aminoglycosides such as gentamicin are not known to affect the cytochrome p450 system. Other p450 inducers include phenytoin and chronic alcohol use. Be aware that broad-spectrum penicillin-based antibiotics such as flucloxacillin

DOI: 10.1201/9781003648222-10

have been linked to inhibiting the effect of warfarin in studies of low-level evidence; close monitoring of INR is thus highly recommended.

Easy mnemonics:

Enzyme Inhibitors SICKFACES.COM	Enzyme Inducers SCRAP GP
Sodium valproate	Sulphonylureas
Cimetidine	Carbamazepine
Ketoconazole	Rifampicin
Fluconazole	Alcohol
Alcohol binge drinking	Phenytoin
Chloramphenicol	Griseofulvin
Erythromycin	Phenobarbital
Sulphonamides	
Omeprazole	
Metronidazole	

3. Management of hyperglycaemia

B. Start intravenous insulin infusion at a rate of 1 U/kg/hour

Diabetic ketoacidosis is a medical emergency that is characterised by the triad of cardinal biochemical features: hyperglycaemia (blood glucose >11), hyperketonaemia (ketonaemia >3 mmol/L and/or ketonuria >2+ on a urine dipstick) and metabolic acidosis (pH <7.3 and HCO_3^- <15). The lack of insulin leads to increased glucose release from glycogen stores, which ultimately leads to an osmotic diuresis. Furthermore, lipolysis and formation of ketone bodies of an acidic profile are produced as a natural compensatory mechanism. A significant proportion of newly diagnosed patients with type 1 diabetes mellitus present with ketoacidosis, although it may present following a stress response to an additional infective or inflammatory condition, induction of medication such as steroids or following trauma, pregnancy or surgery.

Patients often present with vague symptoms such as fatigue, confusion, polyuria and polydipsia, abdominal pain and vomiting. They are likely to have signs of dehydration and potentially hypovolaemic shock on examination. When investigating, one should check blood glucose and ketones, arterial blood gas (ABG) and urine dip, as well as investigate for the source of infection. Consider calculating the anion gap and serum osmolality also.

Rehydration with intravenous fluids is essential but should be done with caution, especially in the elderly, as it can result in fluid overloading. A bolus of normal saline is followed by hourly bags in the initial time period. K^+ supplementation of 40 mmol per litre normal saline is required to keep K^+

between 3.5 and 5.5. Insulin infusion is normally started at a rate of 0.1 U/kg/hour. The patient and blood values are monitored hourly. A urinary catheter is considered in patients with oliguria for fluid balance monitoring. Once blood glucose falls below 14, consider an infusion of dextrose alongside insulin/saline to prevent hypoglycaemia. If the patient normally takes long-acting insulin, continue at the usual dose and time. Involve the diabetic nurses urgently.

4. Skin graft take

A. Adhesion

Skin grafts can be divided into split thickness and full thickness. A full-thickness graft incorporates the epidermis and whole of dermis, while a split-thickness graft contains varying degrees of dermal tissue. The skin graft is taken from a donor site – in the case of a split-thickness skin graft, usually the thigh. Take is a term used to describe graft viability following grafting. There are four steps to a take, and they include adhesion, plasmic inhibition, neo/revascularisation and remodelling. The bed of the recipient site should be optimised to allow take, or else graft failure will occur. The graft take can be affected by local and systemic factors such as haematoma, seroma, poor vascular supply, inadequate wound bed such as exposed bone and steroids. Infection, particularly *Streptococcus* infection, affects adhesion and thus will negatively affect graft take. One must clear infection prior to grafting using local antimicrobial guidelines to aid management.

5. Investigation of hypothyroidism

B. Magnetic resonance imaging (MRI) of the brain

The most common cause of hypothyroidism worldwide is iodine deficiency. Most cases of hypothyroidism in developed countries are caused by auto-immune thyroid disease such as Hashimoto's and thyroid failure following ^{131}I or surgical treatment of thyrotoxicosis. Patients often present with fatigue, depression, constipation, cold intolerance and occasionally carpal tunnel syndrome. On examination one may find bradycardia, dry skin, hair loss and weight gain.

Hypothyroidism usually results from an intrinsic disorder of the thyroid gland, in which the thyroid function test shows a low serum T_4 and elevated thyroid-stimulating hormone (TSH) level; this is known as primary hypothyroidism. In this case, however, the low serum T_4 and low TSH level suggest central hypothyroidism (secondary hypothyroidism), which warrants magnetic resonance imaging (MRI) of the brain to visualise the hypothalamic–pituitary axis.

6. Sickle cell disease

D. Rehydration and analgesia

This patient is having a sickle cell crisis. Such events are triggered by cold weather, infection and dehydration typically. A sickle cell crisis can involve several different pathological mechanisms, including vaso-occlusive, sequestration, haemolytic and aplastic crisis. The mainstay of treatment is analgesia, rehydration and oxygen therapy. Joints involved in sickle crises are prone to infection, particularly *Salmonella,* and therefore a low threshold is required before starting antibiotics. Sickle cell disease is more common in Afro-Caribbean populations and has many forms, of which sickle cell anaemia (Hbss) is the most severe. It is caused by a mutation in the beta-globin gene and a change of amino acid from glutamine to valine in codon 6. Patients with sickle cell trait/carriers are largely asymptomatic. The disease leads to red blood cells occluding blood vessels and being broken down prematurely, rendering the patient anaemic and at risk of stroke, blindness, renal failure, pigmented gallstones, bowel ischaemia and priapism. Long-term management of these patients must be undertaken in specialist centres, and management options include psychological support, lifestyle advice, prophylactic antibiotics, up-to-date immunisations, blood transfusions, hydroxyurea and bone marrow transplants. Unfortunately, 50% of patients die before 40 years.

7. Skin cancer

B. They readily metastasise to bone

Basal cell carcinoma (BCC) is the most common skin cancer arising from the basal cells of the epidermis. They are primarily locally infiltrative; however, with time they may metastasise. They typically develop in sun-exposed areas and are more commonly seen in those with Fitzpatrick type 1 skin, older people and patients suffering from Gorlin syndrome – an autosomal dominant condition characterised by multiple BCC and odontogenic keratocysts. Management is commonly with excision with 4-mm margins and histological assessment, with further excision if margins are involved. Other treatment options include topical creams such as imiquimod cream or 5-fluorouracil, cryotherapy and curette or cauterisation.

8. Skin manifestations of systemic disease

C. Dermatitis herpetiformis

Dermatitis herpetiformis is a blistering, intensely itchy rash that develops on the extensor surfaces. It is associated with coeliac disease and is treated with dapsone and a gluten-free diet. Other cutaneous features of gastrointestinal disease include:

Malabsorption	→ Ichthyosis (dry, scaly skin), eczema, oedema
Liver disease	→ Jaundice, spider naevi, palmar erythema, leukonychia
Renal failure	→ Itching, half-white and half-red nails
Crohn's disease	→ Perianal abscess, fistulae, skin tags, aphthous ulcers
Ulcerative colitis	→ Erythema nodosum, pyoderma gangrenosum
Sarcoidosis	→ Erythema nodosum, lupus pernio (purple indurated lesions)

Acrodermatitis enteropathica is a rare inherited defect of zinc malabsorption. Features develop during weaning and include a perianal and oral red, scaly, pustular rash; failure to thrive; diarrhoea; and poor wound healing. Oral hairy leucoplakia is a white rash that develops along the sides of the tongue that cannot be rubbed off (unlike *Candida*). It is caused by the Epstein–Barr virus infection and may be a sign of underlying human immunodeficiency virus (HIV) infection. Linea nigra is a dark line of pigmentation running down from the umbilicus that is a normal skin feature of pregnancy.

9. Hepatic haemangioma

D. No treatment necessary

Hepatic haemangiomas are common benign tumours of the liver present in 3–7% of the population. The majority do not cause any symptoms and are incidental findings. If a haemangioma is especially large or causing obstruction, it may be considered for surgical removal; otherwise, no treatment is required.

10. Oxygen therapy

A. 28%

The arterial blood gas (ABG) of this patient shows that he has type 2 respiratory failure with respiratory acidosis. The administration of high-flow oxygen will lead to worsening of the hypercapnic respiratory failure. In this situation, the oxygen therapy should be started at 28% or 24% using a Venturi mask (controlled delivery) and modified depending on oxygen saturation and subsequent blood gas results. If oxygen administration results in failure of oxygenation or worsening hypercapnia, then non-invasive ventilation should be considered. When managing patients with increased oxygen demands, one must consider the oxygen cascade. This is a natural process by which the PO_2 will decrease as we take air in from the atmosphere to the mitochondria. If one has reduced ventilation due to an exacerbation of COPD, then this decline will be dramatically exaggerated, and thus one needs to supplement the patient with O_2 to prevent the tissues becoming hypoxic. This is summarised by Henry's law in that the amount of dissolved gas in a liquid, i.e. blood is proportional to the partial pressure to which it exerts.

11. Polycystic kidney disease

A. Bladder diverticuli

Cerebral aneurysms are associated with polycystic kidney disease, and thus the risk of subarachnoid haemorrhage is increased. For this reason, blood pressure should be monitored carefully and hypertension treated swiftly. Hepatic cysts and pancreatic cysts are associated, but only occasionally can be large and symptomatic (dull ache, acute pain caused by rupture or obstructive symptoms such as obstructive jaundice). Mitral valve prolapse and mitral regurgitation are also linked. Bladder diverticuli are usually secondary to urinary outflow obstruction and can become infected due to stagnant urine or obstruction of their outlet. They are not associated with polycystic kidney disease.

12. Hip pain

E. Iliotibial band syndrome

The iliotibial band is a continuation of the tensor fascia lata and inserts into the lateral tibial condyle. It supports flexion of the hip and the knee. It is commonly irritated and inflamed if one overexerts themselves. It causes pain in the hip radiating to the knee and is particularly painful when placing weight on the affected limb. As the patient is well and does not describe any fever, weight loss or nocturnal pain, infection and malignancy are unlikely. She is unlikely to have osteoarthritis at 28 years of age, and there is no family history or systemic signs of rheumatoid arthritis. Management is with rest, ice, elevation and thorough warming up and down during exercise.

13. Hyperbilirubinaemia

B. Gilbert's disease

Gilbert's disease (or Gilbert's syndrome) is a benign partial deficiency in the glucuronyl transferase, the enzyme that's required to conjugate bilirubin. People with this condition have a mildly raised non-haemolytic unconjugated hyperbilirubinaemia, especially when they are acutely unwell. The remainder of the liver function tests are unaffected. Often this is picked up on routine screening, although some patients may experience intermittent jaundice. This condition requires no treatment.

Crigler–Najjar syndrome is a very rare autosomal recessive disorder of childhood caused by deficient metabolism of bilirubin. In this disease there is either a total or partial deficiency of hepatic glucuronyl transferase leading to high amounts of unconjugated bilirubin in the serum. Both types present with severe jaundice during the neonatal period and require phototherapy and plasmapheresis to reduce the levels of bilirubin in the serum. A liver transplant may be needed. There is often some development of brain damage by adulthood.

John Fielding Crigler, American paediatrician (b. 1919)

Nicholas Augustin Gilbert, French physician (1858-1927)

Victor Assad Najjar, American paediatrician (b. 1914)

14. Drugs used in cardiac arrest

A. Adrenaline

Adrenaline interacts with alpha- and beta-adrenergic receptors to cause peripheral and splanchnic vasoconstriction, which divert blood away from the skin and gastrointestinal tract to the heart and brain. The net effect is an increase in coronary and cerebral perfusion pressures. Current resuscitation protocols advise that adrenaline is given as a 1-mg intravenous dose of 1:10,000 solution with the third shock and every 3–5 minutes thereafter in shockable arrhythmias (i.e. ventricular fibrillation and pulseless ventricular tachycardia). In non-shockable rhythms (e.g. asystole and pulseless electrical activity), adrenaline should be given at the start of the resuscitation attempt and every 3–5 minutes thereafter. Adrenaline is also available in a 1:1000 solution, which is reserved for use in anaphylaxis, where it is given intramuscularly.

Amiodarone is a membrane-stabilising drug that increases the refractory period of the cardiac cycle. Atropine is an anti-muscarinic drug that blocks the vagal nerve, thus increasing the rate of sinoatrial node and atrioventricular node depolarisation. Magnesium sulphate can be given as a 2-g (8 mmol) intravenous bolus in ventricular fibrillation refractory to defibrillation. Calcium gluconate stabilises the myocardium against the toxic actions of potassium and is used as cardioprotection in hyperkalaemia.

15. Management of thyrotoxicosis

B. Carbimazole therapy

The history and examination suggest a diagnosis of Graves' disease. This is the most common cause of hyperthyroidism and is typically due to thyroid-stimulating immunoglobulins targeting the thyroid-stimulating hormone (TSH) receptors of the thyroid gland. Signs and symptoms are typically lid retraction, ophthalmoplegia and proptosis coupled with agitation, poor sleep, goitre, tachycardia, pre-tibial myxoedema and diarrhoea. Management includes medication, radio-iodine and surgical intervention.

Due to the risks of surgery incorporating possible injury to the recurrent or superior laryngeal nerve, as well as hypoparathyroidism, medication is typically trialled first. Antithyroid drugs such as carbimazole or propylthiouracil are given to the patient for a period of 12–18 months. These drugs reduce the synthesis of new thyroid hormones by inhibiting the iodination of tyrosine. Carbimazole in particular carries a risk of agranulocytosis. Carbimazole is also contraindicated in pregnancy, especially in the first trimester, due to teratogenic effects. Therefore propylthiouracil (PTU) or methimazole are given in the first and second trimesters. Beta-blockers are used to control symptoms of thyrotoxicosis such as atrial fibrillation. If not managed, there is a risk of dry eyes and corneal injury, as well as miscarriage.

16. Haemoptysis

E. Tuberculosis

Lung cancer can commonly cause haemoptysis, but given the patient's age and smoking history, this seems unlikely. Lymphoma can cause night sweats and non-specific malaise and can present in patients of such an age; however, the haemoptysis as a specific symptom must be looked into, and lymphoma is not the most parsimonious diagnosis. *Pneumocystis carinii* pneumonia (PCP) can present with dry cough, fever and breathlessness in immunosuppressed patients, particularly patients with HIV. The haemoptysis and lack of breathlessness as a prominent feature go against the diagnosis. Pulmonary embolism can cause haemoptysis; however, it would be acute in onset and typically feature chest pain and breathlessness.

The insidious onset of haemoptysis with malaise and night sweats in a young person of sub-Saharan origin is highly suggestive of pulmonary tuberculosis (TB). TB is caused by *Mycobacterium tuberculosis*, and it is estimated that 23% of the world's population has latent TB. When one inhales TB from the air, the primary infection is usually dealt with by the host immune system. The infection may be cleared in 80% of the cases, become latent and contained or be spread via the bloodstream to other areas of the body such as the vertebrae and kidneys. Latent TB may re-activate if the body is under stress or immunocompromised. If suspected, multiple sputum cultures should be sent for Ziehl–Nielsen staining and culture and a chest X-ray taken. Bronchoalveolar lavage can be performed if sputum is negative. Anyone presenting with TB should be counselled for hepatitis B and C and HIV testing, as these infections are more common in immunosuppressed patients, and our patient's origin adds weight to this suspicion. Management is typically with isoniazid, rifampicin, ethambutol and pyrazinamide. Monitored compliance aids reduction in drug resistance, and liver and renal function should be monitored throughout treatment.

Tuberculosis, from Latin *tuberculum* = small lump (in reference to the primary lung focus)

17. Arterial blood gases

C. Respiratory acidosis

The pH value shows if the gas is acidotic (<7.35) or alkalotic (>7.45). Next, it must be determined whether the alkalosis or acidosis is due to a metabolic or respiratory cause – this is done by looking at the pCO_2 and bicarbonate levels. Two things must be borne in mind before continuing: 1) carbon dioxide is acidic and bicarbonate is alkaline, and 2) bicarbonate equates to "metabolic" and pCO_2 means "respiratory". Alkalosis can be due to either high bicarbonate ("metabolic alkalosis") or a low pCO_2 ("respiratory alkalosis"). Conversely, acidosis can be caused by either low bicarbonate ("metabolic acidosis") or a high pCO_2 ("respiratory acidosis").

In some cases of blood gas disturbance, the body has time to compensate. In other words, whichever chemical is causing the imbalance is counteracted by the opposite one. For example, if there is a high bicarbonate (metabolic alkalosis), then the pCO_2 starts to increase to raise the acidity and counteract the alkalosis. If compensation is successful, the pH will then return to within the normal range (7.35–7.45), even if the bicarbonate and pCO_2 levels are abnormal.

Respiratory failure is defined as a pO_2 <8.0. Type 1 respiratory failure occurs when there is hypoxia in the presence of a low or normal pCO_2. Type 2 respiratory failure is hypoxia in the presence of a high pCO_2.

In this case, the patient has type 2 respiratory failure (pO_2 < 8.0) with respiratory acidosis (low pH and high pCO_2). From the history the patient appears to be tiring and needs urgent respiratory assessment, which may result in ventilation.

18. Dry eyes

A. Artificial tears

At present her only symptom is persistently dry eyes, which is demonstrated by the positive Schirmer's test (see later). This is keratoconjunctivitis sicca, which in the absence of other rheumatological disease, is primary Sjögren's syndrome.

The main features of Sjögren's syndrome are dry eyes (keratoconjunctivitis sicca) and dry mouth (xerostomia). Other features are corneal ulcers, oral *Candida*, vaginal dryness, dyspareunia and respiratory hoarseness. Diagnosis is with the Schirmer's test: a piece of filter paper 35 mm long is placed under the lower eyelid for 5 minutes – moistening of less than 10 mm indicates reduced tear production and is suggestive of keratoconjunctivitis sicca. Anti-Ro and anti-La antibodies may be present. Treatment is with artificial tears and artificial saliva, as these help symptoms and carry few side effects. Surveillance therefore seems slightly cruel. Tear duct–related interventions are rarely, if at all, indicated. Hydroxychloroquine can improve arthralgia and fatigue in connective tissue disorders, and steroids can be used in persistent salivary gland swelling or neuropathy (which can develop in association with Sjögren's syndrome), but neither are indicated here.

Henrik Sjögren, Swedish ophthalmologist (1899-1986)

19. Management of shortness of breath

C. Give IV 5% dextrose immediately

Anaphylaxis is a life-threatening condition caused by a severe allergic reaction to a certain allergen (e.g. drugs, food, insect stings). This leads to systemic release of immune and inflammatory mediators from basophils and mast cells. It is normally initiated by an IgE-mediated hypersensitivity reaction. Patients present with oedema, urticaria, bronchospasm and/or cardiovascular collapse. Patients should avoid further contact with the allergen. The airway should be maintained, and anaesthetic input should be sought immediately. Oxygen should be provided at a high flow rate. Intramuscular adrenaline (0.5 mL of 1:1000 solution) is given immediately, followed by intravenous antihistamines. There is no evidence for using 5% dextrose for fluid resuscitation, as it quickly redistributes itself out of the intravascular space. The fluid of choice is normal saline or Hartmann's.

20. Shoulder injury

B. Axillary

The axillary nerve is a branch of the posterior cord of the brachial plexus (roots C5–6). It passes through the quadrangular space alongside the posterior humeral circumflex artery and provides motor supply to the deltoid and teres minor and sensory supply to the lateral aspect of the shoulder – the "regimental badge". X-rays have shown this gentleman has obtained an anterior shoulder dislocation with likely axillary nerve injury. Orthopaedic review and urgent reduction are essential. However, reduction should not be attempted if there is a fracture dislocation.

21. Haemophilia

B. VIII

Haemophilia A is an X-linked recessive disorder of coagulation in which the patient cannot synthesise clotting factor VIII due to a gene mutation. Haemophilia B (sometime referred to as Christmas disease) is caused by an inability to synthesise factor IX and is clinically indistinguishable from the much more common haemophilia A. Factors VIII and IX are essential in the intrinsic clotting cascade, meaning that patients with haemophilia have a prolonged activated partial thromboplastin time (APTT). The extrinsic pathway does not require factors VIII or IX and is therefore unaffected by haemophilia – shown by a normal prothrombin time (PT). The bleeding time is also normal. Symptoms usually begin when the patient becomes mobile, i.e. when they begin to crawl or walk. Haemophiliacs typically suffer painful recurrent bleeds into the joints and soft tissues (haemarthrosis), which may eventually lead to crippling arthropathy and neuropathy.

The treatment of haemophilia A is with factor VIII concentrate, either as a regular infusion or when actively bleeding. Patients receiving regular infusions have higher factor VIII levels and a better quality of life but are at higher risk of developing antibodies to the extrinsic factor VIII, which reduces its efficiency. Patients who receive factor VIII only when bleeding are less likely to form antibodies but are at increased risk of bleeding. Patients with mild disease may be treated with desmopressin (DDVAP), which releases factor VIII from internal stores. Factor VIII concentrate should be given prior to invasive procedures such as tooth extraction and surgery. Haemophilia B is treated with factor IX concentrate. It should be noted that many haemophiliacs who received blood products prior to the initiation of the blood screening programme have contracted blood-borne viruses such as HIV and hepatitis C.

Von Willebrand factor (vWF) is a co-factor that binds to and mediates the actions of factor VIII binding to platelets. Inheritance is autosomal dominant in the majority, and the gene is carried on chromosome 12. Replacement in severe disease involves cryoprecipitate or additional factor VIII.

Stephen Christmas was the first person described to have factor IX deficiency (1947–1993). He eventually died from acquired immune deficiency syndrome (AIDS), transmitted via a transfusion. The original case report of Christmas disease was reported in the Christmas edition of the *British Medical Journal* in 1952.

22. Gastrointestinal pathology

B. Crohn's disease

The clinical pictures of inflammatory bowel disease (IBD) can often be similar – classically a young woman with diarrhoea, pain and weight loss. IBD is an umbrella term that encompasses Crohn's disease and ulcerative colitis (UC). The former is only located in the distal colon and can appear indistinguishable from UC (which may affect the entire bowel) except on histology. More specifically, Crohn's typically affects the terminal ileum but can affect any part of the gastrointestinal (GI) tract in skip lesions. The inflammation in Crohn's disease affects the entire thickness of the bowel wall – which is why it more often leads to complications such as fistulas and abscesses – whereas in UC the inflammation primarily affects the mucosa and submucosa, leading to ulcer formation and crypt abscesses. Between ulcers, pseudopolyps can form, which tend to be very friable and bleed easily. The management of Crohn's disease comprises bloods, including C-reactive protein (CRP) and erythrocyte sedimentation rate (ESR) and an abdominal X-ray (AXR) to ensure no toxic megacolon. Steroids, either PO or IV pending severity, are required coupled with rehydration. Long-term management is with steroids or steroid-sparing agents such as azathioprine/infliximab. Fifty percent will require surgery, and there is a risk of short bowel syndrome. Long-term complications include bowel obstruction and/or perforation, malignancy of the bowel and gallbladder and fistulas (colovesical/vagina/cutaneous).

Differentiation in this case from GI tuberculosis (TB) is difficult, as both have a predilection for terminal ileum, but TB is more likely to produce caseating granulomas. It is also noted that in TB, there are transverse ulcerations in comparison to longitudinal ulcers seen in Crohn's. However, in regions endemic for TB or in high-risk patients, a thorough history and high index of suspicion are required, even without the presence of caseating granulomas, and appropriate staining should be undertaken for histological specimens. Irritable bowel syndrome does not cause histological changes.

23. Blood film

B. Megaloblastic anaemia

Leucoerythroblastic anaemia describes the presence of immature cells – myelocytes and normoblasts – in the blood film. This can occur by any process that invades the bone marrow causing inappropriate release of immature cells into the circulation. This can be an infective process (such as tuberculous invasion of the bone marrow), primary bone marrow malignancy or metastatic spread into the marrow.

Megaloblastic anaemia is characterised by a raised mean cell volume caused by a reduction in either folate or vitamin B_{12}. It can be associated with hypothyroidism. It can present with fatigue, dyspnoea, palpitations or peripheral neuropathy and, rarely, with ataxia and falls secondary to subacute combined degeneration of the spinal cord.

24. Lung cancer

B. Metabolic alkalosis, small cell carcinoma

Small cell carcinoma comprises 20% of all lung cancers. Small cell lung carcinoma is known to metastasise early and is usually treated palliatively with chemotherapy (with an 80% mortality rate at 1 year). Patients with small cell carcinoma may present with symptoms of extrapulmonary manifestations such as endocrine syndromes (inappropriate antidiuretic hormone [ADH] secretion and ectopic adrenocorticotropic hormone [ACTH] secretion). This patient presents with a hypokalaemic metabolic alkalosis as a result of hypercortisolism associated with raised ACTH secretion (this may also have caused her diabetes). Hypokalaemia is responsible for myopathy, as characterised by weakness in both lower limbs. Lung cancer can be split into small cell (20%) and non–small cell carcinoma (80%). It often presents with chronic cough, haemoptysis and/or dyspnoea. It may also present as a slowly resolving pneumonia or metastatic symptom such as a seizure or bone pain. One must investigate with a chest X-ray, biopsy and a CT scan. Management is based on histology, but generally speaking, non–small cell tumours are managed with surgical resection in the early stages followed by chemoradiotherapy +/– targeted monoclonal antibody therapy. Small cell cancer is usually treated with chemotherapy due to early metastatic activity.

25. Cavernous sinus lesions

D. III, IV, VI and ophthalmic and maxillary division of V

The cavernous sinus lies lateral to the sella turcica. Cranial nerve II (the optic nerve) passes through the optic foramen, medial and superior to the superior orbital fissure, and so does not run through the cavernous sinus. The nerves that do run through the cavernous sinus are those responsible for controlling eye movements (III, IV and VI), as well as the ophthalmic and maxillary division of the V nerve (trigeminal). Also passing is the venous plexus and carotid artery along with its associated sympathetic fibres. Clinically therefore, cavernous sinus pathology presents with a complete ophthalmoplegia of the affected side (often both sides are affected) and a loss of sensation on the affected side in the distribution of the ophthalmic and maxillary nerves. One may also present with proptosis, chemosis and Horner's syndrome. Causative pathologies include cavernous sinus thrombosis (often caused by spread of infection from the nasal mucosa or from a facial pustule), meningioma, pituitary tumours, metastatic cancer and, as the carotid artery runs through the cavernous sinus, carotid aneurysms and carotid-cavernous fistula. MRI is usually the investigation of choice, with treatment based on underlying pathology.

Cavernous, from Latin *cavernosus* = cavity

26. Cognitive impairment

D. Lewy body dementia

Frontotemporal dementia is rare and usually presents with personality change and disinhibition, with a sparing of memory function early on in the disease. Of those with motor neurone disease, 5–10% also get frontotemporal dementia. Vascular dementia occurs with multiple transient ischaemic attacks (TIAs) and strokes, and while this patient is a smoker, there is no history of strokes or TIAs and no neurological deficit on examination suggestive of a stroke. Korsakoff psychosis is characterised by severe impairment of episodic memory function – patients are unable to form new episodic memories and have impaired access to old episodic memories and therefore are liable to confabulate. It is caused by mamillary body damage, normally secondary to untreated Wernicke's encephalopathy (associated with chronic alcohol excess), although it can be secondary to hypoxic brain damage or central nervous system (CNS) infection. Depressive pseudo-dementia presents similarly to Alzheimer's disease and is a common cause of misdiagnosis. It features depressed mood and anxiety, and lack of self-confidence can lead to an apparent short-term memory deficit, although with encouragement and close examination, the memory deficit disappears.

Lewy body dementia is the second most common dementia after Alzheimer's disease. Characteristic features include day-to-day fluctuating levels of cognitive functioning, visual hallucinations, sleep disturbance, transient loss of consciousness, recurrent falls and parkinsonian features (tremor, hypokinesia, rigidity and postural instability). Although people with Lewy body dementia are prone to hallucinations, antipsychotics should be avoided, as they precipitate severe parkinsonism in 60%. A Lewy body is an abnormality of the cytoplasm found within a neurone containing various proteins and granular material. Lewy bodies are found in the cerebral cortex in patients with Lewy body dementia, and they are also found in patients with Parkinson's disease.

27. Complications of bone marrow transplant

B. Chronic graft-versus-host disease

Graft-versus-host disease (GVHD) can occur either acutely or chronically following any form of transplant. It is a T-cell–driven response of the transplanted graft to the host. The severity can vary from self-limiting irritation to life-threatening disease. This can present with a myriad of symptoms but most commonly skin, liver and gastrointestinal tract manifestations. Treatment is twofold: symptomatic and immunosuppressive. Prevention of GVHD is targeted with immunosuppressant drugs such as tacrolimus or T-cell–depleted grafts; however, there is a balance between prevention of GVHD and cancer treatment.

28. Diagnosis of abdominal pain

A. Fitz-Hugh–Curtis syndrome

Fitz-Hugh–Curtis syndrome is a rare complication of pelvic inflammatory disease (PID), where ascending disease results in inflammation of the connective tissue around the liver (Glisson's capsule). It is often caused by gonococcal or chlamydial infection. It is predominantly a disease of women and only rarely affects men. Diagnosis is through the identification of PID and the exclusion of other diseases, including pancreatitis. Liver function tests are usually normal. Treatment is with antibiotics as for PID. Other complications of PID include chronic pelvic pain, ectopic pregnancy and malignancy of the upper genital tract.

Thomas Fitz-Hugh Jr, American physician (1894–1963)

Arthur Curtis, American gynaecologist (1881–1955)

29. Diagnosis of cough

D. *Pneumocystis jirovecii*

Pneumocystis jirovecii pneumonia is the most common AIDS-defining illness. In HIV-positive adults, the greatest risk factor for developing *Pneumocystis* pneumonia (PCP) is a CD4 count of below 200 cells/mm^3. The incidence of PCP has reduced significantly with the use of highly active antiretroviral therapy (HAART) and routine primary prophylaxis in those with a CD4 count of less than 200 cells/mm^3. Most cases of PCP occur in patients who are unaware of their HIV infection or do not use HAART or PCP prophylaxis due to intolerance or non-compliance. PCP could also affect patients who are on chronic immunosuppressive therapy, solid organ transplant recipients and bone marrow transplant recipients. Patients present with a non-productive dry cough, dyspnoea, weight loss, fatigue and possibly pleuritic chest pain, which is uncommon in PCP without a pneumothorax. Chest examination is usually unremarkable. Chest X-ray findings include bilateral symmetrical interstitial infiltrates with perihilar reticular opacities, lobar consolidation, nodular lesions, pneumothorax and pneumomediastinum, although findings can be normal. Treatment involves co-trimoxazole (a combination of trimethoprim and sulfamethoxazole) for a 3-week duration and corticosteroids in severe cases. Patients with respiratory compromise require admission to the intensive care unit for mechanical ventilation.

30. Palpitations

E. Phaeochromocytoma

Phaeochromocytoma is a rare tumour arising from the catecholamine-producing chromaffin cells from the adrenal medulla. Approximately 90% arise in the adrenal gland, and the remainder are extra-adrenal in origin. Most of these tumours are sporadic in origin, but about 10% may manifest from a hereditary syndrome such as multiple endocrine neoplasia type 2, Von Hippel–Lindau syndrome and neurofibromatosis. The patient presents with episodic palpitations, headache, excessive sweating, pallor and paroxysmal hypertension. Some present with a complication of hypertension, e.g.

stroke, myocardial infarction, hypertensive retinopathy and accelerated-phase hypertension. The diagnosis is obtained by increased levels of urinary catecholamines, metanephrines and normetanephrines. Treatment options include medical management, which aims to block the effects of catecholamine excess by controlling hypertension using alpha-receptor blockers, or surgical removal of the tumour. An alpha-blocker is given pre-operatively to prevent a sympathetic surge when the tumour is manipulated surgically.

31. Diagnosis of neurological dysfunction

D. Subacute combined degeneration of the cord

Subacute combined degeneration of the cord is caused by vitamin B_{12} deficiency. Her malnourishment and poverty are the likely cause of this. Note the conjunctival pallor – B_{12} deficiency also causes macrocytic megaloblastic anaemia. In addition to the consequence of anaemia in B_{12} deficiency, psychiatric disturbance may also ensue. The pathology – in this case demyelination – predominantly affects the lateral corticospinal tract and posterior columns. The clinical picture of a subacute onset of mixed upper and lower motor neurone lower limb weakness and loss of vibration, proprioception and light touch is classic. Prompt investigation and treatment are required, as response to B_{12} supplementation is inversely proportional to the severity of symptoms.

32. Diagnosis of skin lesions

C. Irregular pigment network

Erythema of the border when looking at a pigmented lesion can raise suspicion that it may be malignant melanoma; however, seborrhoeic keratoses can become inflamed, and this is therefore a non-specific characteristic. A granular surface is a typical feature of seborrhoeic keratoses when inspected up close. A "stuck-on" appearance is again typical for seborrhoeic keratoses and does not require dermoscopy to spot. Telangiectasia of the skin surface is far more typical of basal cell carcinomas. An irregular pigment network may be highly important in differentiating a malignant melanoma from a benign pigmented lesion and may be picked up by dermoscopy – a flat, low-resolution glass is placed directly on the area of interest to magnify the appearance of the skin. When assessing a potential melanoma, one must consider ABCDE – asymmetry, irregular borders, colour variability, diameter >7 mm and evolving and elevated from the skin.

33. Malignant melanoma

D. Invasive depth

Staging depends upon the thickness: stage 1 has tumour <1 mm depth; stage 2, 1–2 mm; stage 3, 2–4 mm; and stage 4, >4 mm depth. Breslow thickness is measured from the granular layer of the epidermis. Other useful prognosticators explored during histological assessment include ulceration and mitotic rate.

Alexander Breslow, American pathologist (1928-1980)

34. Electrocardiogram

C. Provide immediate cardioversion

The patient is stable and so does not need immediate cardioversion. One should look for the cause and treat accordingly. Tricyclic antidepressants (e.g. imipramine, amitriptyline); type 1a antiarrhythmics (e.g. quinidine, procainamide); antibiotics (fluoroquinolones and macrocodes); and hypokalaemia/hypomagnesaemia are known to cause acquired torsade de pointes secondary to prolonged QT. Congenital causes include Romana–Ward and Jevell and Lange–Nielsen syndromes. Between reviewing the drug chart and looking up this patient's most recent serum electrolytes, you would be wise to inform your seniors and a cardiologist. The patient should be linked to a cardiac monitor. It also would be wise to ensure the crash trolley is ready for use.

35. Diagnosis of chest infection

E. Severe community-acquired pneumonia

There is no history of choking or aspiration or any at-risk conditions (e.g. epileptic fits, Parkinson's disease, alcoholism) to suggest aspiration pneumonia. Whilst the blunting of the costophrenic angle suggests an effusion, it sounds small and is unlikely to represent an empyema – it could be a parapneumonic effusion or could be unrelated. Whilst he was in hospital for a hernia repair, this was likely a short visit, and it was 2 months ago, after which he has been well, so it is not hospital-acquired pneumonia. Community-acquired pneumonia is graded using the CURB-65 score: patients score from 0 to 5, picking up points for (1) confusion (new AMTS < 8); (2) urea > 7 mmol/L; (3) respiratory rate > 30/min; (4) blood pressure < 90 systolic or < 60 diastolic mmHg; or (5) age > 65. A score of 0–1 is mild, 2 is moderate and 3 or more is severe. Our patient scored at least 3 for his age, new confusion and a respiratory rate >30 and so has a severe community-acquired pneumonia. Hospital guidelines for antibiotic use in pneumonia vary across the country due to differing organisms and sensitivities, but severity of pneumonia and the community/hospital distinction are used to guide initial empirical therapies. This patient will require a full septic screen and need to be commenced on IV antibiotics and high-flow oxygen immediately.

36. Emergency management

B. Intramuscular benzylpenicillin and call ambulance

This patient has the clinical features of meningitis with septicaemia (neck stiffness in association with general illness and a non-blanching purpuric rash). It is essential that this patient is given antibiotics as soon as possible and admitted to a high-dependency unit. If the patient is seen in the community, she should be given an intramuscular dose of benzylpenicillin whilst transport to hospital is being arranged. Once in hospital, the patient will require intravenous antibiotics (e.g. cefotaxime) for at least 7 days in addition to supportive measures. Risks of meningitis can be divided into acute (multiorgan failure secondary to sepsis) or chronic (seizures, intellectual disturbance, hearing and visual impairment).

37. Investigation of shortness of breath

D. Spirometry

With his history of smoking, it is highly likely that this patient has developed chronic obstructive pulmonary disease (COPD). The diagnosis of COPD requires spirometry. A post-bronchodilator $FEV_1/FVC < 70\%$ confirms the diagnosis, and depending on the value of FEV_1 of <80%, severity staging can be undertaken. A low peak flow is consistent with COPD, but it is not a specific test, as it could underestimate the severity of airflow obstruction and is unable to differentiate obstructive and restrictive disorders. Chest X-ray is useful in excluding other lung pathology and might detect bullae associated with COPD.

38. Diagnosis of chest pain

B. Gastro-oesophageal reflux disease

Differentiating gastro-oesophageal reflux disease (GORD) from a cardiac cause of pain can be extremely difficult. In this case the salient feature is that the pain occurs on lying down to go to sleep. Although in unstable angina this may occur, you would also expect a patient to report pain on increased exertion as well. A glyceryl trinitrite (GTN) spray may relieve both GORD and angina, as the nitrates cause smooth muscle relaxation in the oesophagus as well as coronary arteries, reducing oesophageal spasms. Some GORD patients even get referred to respiratory physicians with chronic cough or exacerbation of asthma.

GORD is associated with obesity, smoking, alcohol, hernias and pregnancy. Patients generally present with intermittent pain, or heartburn, which may be related to lifestyle factors such as large meals or alcohol. Medications such as steroids and non-steroidal anti-inflammatory drugs (NSAIDs) can also contribute and should be reviewed. Endoscopy is not usually indicated for the diagnosis in young, otherwise healthy patients; however, urgent referrals should be considered in anyone over the age of 55 years with new-onset symptoms or warning signs of weight loss, gastrointestinal (GI) bleeding or anaemia. Management of dyspepsia is by modification of lifestyle factors, including weight loss, and pharmacological treatment with proton pump inhibitors. Tests for *Helicobacter pylori* and treatment are provided accordingly. Potential complications of long-standing reflux are the development of Barrett's oesophagus and the formation of strictures or even adenocarcinoma. It must also be noted that such patients have poor-quality sleep and thus are at risk of associated sequelae.

39. Hypoxia

A. Check her fluid balance chart

This woman is probably suffering from pulmonary oedema, which is easily caused or exacerbated by over-administration of intravenous fluids. At such low saturations, an arterial blood gas analysis should be undertaken, as it is superior to pulse oximetry (which can be erroneous at low saturations) and will also allow you to monitor carbon dioxide levels and metabolic compensation. If highly suspicious of pulmonary oedema, sit the patient up, and administer high-flow O_2 and IV furosemide therapy. Don't be hesitant to start do not attempt cardiopulmonary resuscitation (DNACPR) discussions in such situations after the patient has been stabilised.

40. Management of hypothermia

C. Intravenous lorazepam

Myxoedema coma is a rare presentation of extreme hypothyroidism. It is a medical emergency, and treatment should be initiated before confirmation of the diagnosis. Patients present with a depressed level of consciousness, low body temperature and convulsions, as well as bradycardia and hypotension. An intravenous bolus of triiodothyronine (T_3) is given. Warm blankets could be used to increase body temperature. The thyroid failure should be assumed to be secondary to hypothalamus or pituitary disease, and IV hydrocortisone should be given before thyroid function tests become available. High-flow oxygen is given to patients with low oxygen saturations. IV fluids should also be administrated.

41. Diagnosis of diabetes

E. Urine ketones

In patients with presenting symptoms suggesting diabetes mellitus, the diagnosis could be confirmed by fasting glucose ≥ 7.0 mmol/L or random glucose ≥ 11.1 mmol/L. In asymptomatic patients, two samples are required to confirm diabetes. An oral glucose tolerance test is indicated when fasting plasma glucose is within 6.1–6.9 mmol/L or random plasma glucose is within 7.8–11.0 mmol/L (levels suggestive of impaired glucose tolerance). HbA1C >48 or 6.5% can be used to diagnose diabetes and gives an indication for glycaemic control over 3 months. (*Of note*: HbA1C is unreliable in those with a shortened red blood cell life span such as in sickle cell anaemia. Urine ketones are not diagnostic of diabetes mellitus and may also be raised in malnutrition.)

42. Medication review

D. Propranolol

It should be noted that (1) beta-blockers are contraindicated in asthma, a very common co-morbidity; (2) beta-adrenergic receptors stimulate the fight-or-flight response; (3) beta-1 receptors increase cardiac contractility, heart rate and renin release; (4) beta-2 receptors relax bronchial smooth muscle (the target of salbutamol); and (5) beta-3 receptors instigate lipolysis in adipose tissue. Propranolol is non-selective (because it blocks both beta-1 and beta-2 receptors) and thus should not be used in asthmatic patients.

43. Side effects of methotrexate

B. Alcohol should be absolutely avoided whilst taking methotrexate

Methotrexate is used in the treatment of certain cancers, as well as autoimmune conditions such as psoriasis and rheumatoid arthritis. It acts by inhibiting dihydrofolate reductase and thus DNA and RNA synthesis. It also downregulates T-cell activity. A baseline chest X-ray is indeed taken when starting methotrexate, as pulmonary fibrosis can be a side effect of long-term methotrexate use. Liver function aberrations are the most common side effect and can lead to hepatic fibrosis soon after starting methotrexate. Therefore, liver function tests are initially monitored weekly, followed by fortnightly and then every 4–6 weeks. Whilst alcohol intake above 12 units per week can increase the risk of liver damage, it is permissible for patients to have a small amount of alcohol, though it is advised against. Neutropenia and myelosuppression are risks, and therefore the full blood count is monitored along with liver function tests. Methotrexate blocks the action of folate and therefore is contraindicated in pregnancy due to the risk of neural tube defects.

44. Raised intracranial pressure

E. Transient bilateral visual loss

Jaw claudication is a sign of temporal arteritis. Kernig's sign (with the patient lying on their back with their hip flexed and the knee extension causing pain) is a sign of meningism, as the manoeuvre stretches the nerve roots in the leg, whose sheaths are continuous with the meninges of the central nervous system. On lying down, gravity causes an increase in intracranial pressure, so it would be expected that the symptoms would get worse. Increased intracranial pressure could either cause or be caused by hydrocephalus, and this can compress the optic nerve (increased fluid in the nerve sheath). A late sign therefore may be episodes of transient bilateral visual loss provoked by postural change, e.g. lying down. Fundoscopy should be conducted, looking for papilloedema. Finally, as increased intracranial pressure is considered, lumbar puncture is contraindicated, as it may provoke transforaminal herniation and thus cardiorespiratory compromise by medullary compression.

45. Bronchial carcinoma

D. Squamous cell carcinoma

Lung carcinoma is the most common cause of cancer death in men and women in the UK. It is strongly associated with cigarette smoking, which is thought to be responsible for more than 90% of cases of lung carcinoma. Squamous cell carcinoma is the most common histological type, which accounts for about 35% of bronchial carcinoma. Patients with hypercalcaemia are most likely to have squamous cell carcinoma, as it stimulates the secretion of parathyroid hormone–like peptides, which causes a rise in blood calcium levels by osteolysis in bone and promotes the reabsorption of calcium from renal tubules. The hypercalcaemia should be managed with aggressive fluids and bisphosphonates and then referral made to the oncology team.

46. Neurological dysfunction

C. Median nerve

The nerve roots can be ruled out, as C6 supplies the thumb and index finger, and C8 supplies the fourth and little finger. The ulnar nerve supplies sensation to the medial half of the fourth finger and the entire fifth finger. The radial nerve supplies sensation to a patch of skin on the radial side of the back of the hand. The sensory distribution described is supplied by the median nerve. The thenar muscles are supplied by the median nerve, hence the thenar wasting and weakness of thumb abduction (abductor pollicis brevis). The shooting pains and lack of any history of trauma would make carpal tunnel syndrome the most likely cause.

The carpal tunnel is bound to the flexor retinaculum or transverse carpal ligament overlying the carpal bones. Running through it are the tendons of the flexor digitorum superficialis and profundus, as well as the flexor pollicis longus and the median nerve. Carpal tunnel syndrome is more common in women, during pregnancy and with certain medical conditions such as rheumatoid arthritis, acromegaly and hypothyroidism. Patients experience tingling and numbness in the radial three and a half digits, which may be followed by wasting of the thenar eminence (supplied by the median nerve). Clinical tests that help confirm carpal tunnel syndrome include Tinel's test (tapping over the median nerve at the wrist reproduces symptoms) and Phalen's test (symptoms are reproduced by holding the wrist palmar flexed for 1 minute). Nerve conduction studies and ultrasound can aid the diagnosis. Management options include physiotherapy and a nocturnal splint, steroid injections and release of the transverse carpal ligament.

Jules Tinel, French neurologist (1879-1952)

George Phalen, American orthopaedic surgeon (1911-1998)

47. Diagnosis of rheumatoid arthritis

E. Ulnar deviation of one or more fingers for more than 6 weeks

All of the clinical features are suggestive of rheumatoid arthritis; the important difference, however, is that ulnar deviation of the fingers is a late manifestation that occurs due to subluxation at the metacarpophalangeal joints, which only happens after significant irreversible joint damage. Ideally any diagnostic criteria would focus on early diagnosis so that disease-modifying antirheumatic drugs (DMARDs) can be started promptly. Rheumatoid arthritis commonly causes morning stiffness (in osteoarthritis, stiffness is typically worse after movement at the affected joints), and due to the systemic nature of the cause, diffuse and sometimes symmetrical joint involvement can be seen, whereas osteoarthritis is commonly related to physical wear and tear and thus can be localised and is not necessarily symmetrical.

The diagnosis of rheumatoid arthritis is made using the American Rheumatism Association criteria, requiring four of the following seven factors to be present:

1. Morning stiffness > 1 hour for more than 6 weeks
2. Arthritis of hand joints (wrist, metacarpophalangeal [MCP], proximal interphalangeal [PIP]) for more than 6 weeks
3. Arthritis of three or more joint areas for more than 6 weeks
4. Symmetric arthritis for more than 6 weeks
5. Rheumatoid nodules
6. Characteristic X-ray findings
7. Positive rheumatoid factor

The four characteristic X-ray findings of rheumatoid arthritis are soft tissue swelling, narrowed joint space, juxta-articular erosions and subluxation. Anti-CCP antibody has higher specificity than rheumatoid factor for rheumatoid arthritis.

48. Statistics

D. 83%

The specificity is the ability of an investigation to detect a truly negative test result.

$$\text{Specificity} = \text{number of true negatives/(number of true negatives + number of false positives)} \times 100$$

$$\text{In this case} = 25\ (25 + 5) \times 100 = 83\%$$

49. Sepsis syndromes

B. Septic shock

Septicaemia describes the state of having an organism in the blood, which this woman has; however, this does not fully describe the situation. Systemic inflammatory response syndrome (SIRS) is defined as having two or more of the following four criteria: pulse >90 beats per minute, temperature <36°C or >38°C, respiratory rate >20 breaths/minute, $PaCO_2$ <4.3 kPa (hyperventilatory hypocapnia) or white cell count <4 or >12 10^9/L.

This woman has SIRS, as evidenced by her pulse, temperature and respiratory rate. The combination of SIRS and septicaemia is known as sepsis. Severe sepsis is when a septic patient is showing signs of organ hypoperfusion – for instance, oliguria (kidney hypoperfusion), confusion (brain hypoperfusion) or serum lactate >4 (muscle hypoperfusion). This woman is oliguric and confused. Shock means hypotension, and septic shock is defined as sepsis with refractory hypotension (i.e. hypotension persevering in spite of fluid resuscitation), which applies to this patient. She should be escalated to a senior, as she may need high-dependency/intensive care unit (HDU/ICU) intervention.

50. Nephrotic syndrome

D. >3.5 g of protein lost in the urine over 24 hours

Nephrotic syndrome is a triad of proteinuria, hypoalbuminaemia and oedema. The proteinuria is classically quantified as more than 3.5 g in 24 hours. When phaeochromocytoma is suspected, 72-hour urine collection is performed to look for urinary metanephrines and other catecholamine metabolites. Quantification of proteinuria, rather than simply dipstick testing, is important, as both hypoalbuminaemia and proteinuria are non-specific and can be present in important clinical differentials (cardiac failure can feature mild proteinuria, and liver failure can result in hypoalbuminaemia – both cause oedema and fatigue). A newer test that can spare the hassle of 24-hour urine collection is the urine protein: creatinine ratio, which can reliably predict the amount of protein excreted in the urine over 24 hours from a random urine sample. Nephrotic syndrome is most commonly caused by glomerulonephritides, and so further testing should look for other features of glomerulonephritis and causes thereof (renal autoimmune screen, serum and urine electrophoresis, urine microscopy). Such patients are at risk of blood clots and infections. Adults with nephrotic syndrome should get a renal biopsy to further elucidate the cause; in children, minimal-change glomerulonephritis is the most common cause, and this normally reverses with steroids; hence biopsy can be avoided unless there are other concerning features or there is little response to steroids. Management typically involves sound nutrition with the help of a dietician, diuretics and immunosuppressants. Hyperlipidaemia is treated with statins, whilst low-molecular-weight heparin and antibiotics are used for signs of venous thromboembolism and infection, respectively.

Practice paper 6: Questions

1. Amenorrhoea

A 16-year-old female attends her GP complaining of a persistent lack of periods (primary amenorrhoea). She has a short stature, low-set ears and broad, square-shaped chest. She has a short fourth metacarpal. There is radioradial delay on examination.

What would the most appropriate diagnostic test be in this case?

A Growth hormone level
B Karyotype analysis
C Magnetic resonance angiography
D Thyroid function test
E Ultrasound of the ovaries

2. Myasthenia gravis

Which of the following investigation findings would you NOT expect in myasthenia gravis?

A Decrementing response on electromyography
B Hyperplasia of the thymus gland or thymoma on computed tomography (CT) of the chest
C Positive acetylcholine receptor antibodies
D Rimmed vacuoles on muscle biopsy
E Tensilon test reduces weakness

3. Hyperkalaemia

A 78-year-old man admitted with severe sepsis secondary to a chest infection develops worsening acute renal failure. An arterial blood gas reading, other than showing metabolic acidosis, also reveals a potassium level of 7.2 mmol/L. You ask the nurse for an electrocardiogram (ECG).

Which of the following changes is NOT associated with hyperkalaemia?

A Broadening of the QRS complex
B Deepening Q-waves
C Flattening of the P-waves
D Tented T-waves
E Ventricular fibrillation

DOI: 10.1201/9781003648222-11

4. Myocardial infarction

A 75-year-old man with known heart failure presents to the hospital complaining of chest pain 1 week ago and feeling unwell since. The working diagnosis is likely late-presentation myocardial infarction. He is now haemodynamically stable on the ward. A random troponin level is raised. Which investigation will confirm your diagnosis?

A 24-hour ECG
B Exercise ECG
C Troponin level at 48 hours
D Nuclear studies of the myocardium
E None of the above

5. Pruritus

A 45-year-old woman presents with a 5-month history of worsening generalised itching. There is nothing remarkable in the woman's medical history, and there is no sign of any skin lesion or inflammatory disorder of the skin. You take some blood tests for a pruritus screen.

Which of the following tests would NOT reveal a cause for pruritus and thus is NOT indicated?

A Electrolytes
B Full blood count
C Iron studies
D Thyroid function tests
E Urea

6. Seizures

Which of the following symptoms would NOT be caused by complex partial seizures?

A Déjà-vu
B Fumbling or rubbing, slightly odd limb movements
C Shooting/electric shock–like pains in the limbs
D Smell and/or taste hallucinations
E Subtly impaired conscious level

7. Spinal cord compression

A 70-year-old woman with a background of bowel cancer, which was resected 2 years ago, presents with a 3-week history of back pain, progressive clumsiness and heaviness of the legs with paraesthesia. On examination, the arms are normal, but there is weakness throughout the legs, brisk reflexes, upgoing plantars and diminished sensation bilaterally up to the belly button.

Where is the lesion likely to be?

A C5
B L2
C T8
D T10
E T12

8. Sepsis

A 50-year-old man being treated for inoperable gastric cancer with chemotherapy presents with a sore throat and cough. On examination, he has a temperature of 38.2°C.

Which of the following statements indicates the most severe life-threatening illness?

A Cough of >2 weeks' duration
B Neutrophils >15 × 10^9/L
C Neutrophils <0.5 × 10^9/L
D Severe vomiting
E Weight loss

9. Radiographic changes in ankylosing spondylitis

A 22-year-old man with a family history of psoriasis attends clinic complaining of lower back and buttock pains on and off for the past 6 months. This is worse in the mornings and associated with stiffness.

Which of the following findings on MRI would be first to appear and thus diagnostic of early ankylosing spondylitis?

A Bamboo spine
B Fusion of the sacroiliac joints
C Osteophyte formation
D Sacroiliitis
E Syndesmophyte formation

10. Management of toxicity

An 80-year-old woman is admitted to hospital with a fracture of the right neck of the femur. She became drowsy with a respiratory rate of 8/min after a dose of intravenous morphine. There are pinpoint pupils on examination.

What should you do?

A Give intravenous flumazenil
B Give intravenous magnesium sulphate
C Give intravenous *N*-acetylcysteine
D Give intravenous naloxone
E Give intravenous sodium bicarbonate

11. Squamous cell carcinoma

Which statement is FALSE about squamous cell carcinoma?

A Curettage is the first line of management
B Sun exposure is a risk factor
C They are ill-defined lesions and often ulcerate
D They are more common in kidney transplant patients
E They can metastasise to lymph nodes

12. Management of urinary tract infection

A 28-year-old pregnant woman has a routine mid-stream urine sample for dipstick testing and microscopy culture and sensitivities. She is asymptomatic.

Which of the following results warrants a course of antibiotics?

A Leukocyte esterase negative, nitrites negative
B Leukocyte esterase negative, nitrites negative, but >10⁵/mL Gram-negative rods on microscopy
C Leukocyte esterase negative, nitrites positive
D Leukocyte esterase positive, nitrites negative
E Leukocyte esterase positive, nitrites positive

13. Side effects of anti-tuberculous medication

A 35-year-old homeless man diagnosed with new tuberculosis 1 month previously started on treatment presents with loss of colour vision.

Which of the following medications is responsible?

A Ethambutol
B Isoniazid
C Pyrazinamide
D Rifampicin
E Streptomycin

14. Hypothyroidism

A 64-year-old woman with known heart disease presents to her GP with weight gain, weakness and bilateral leg swelling. On examination she has slow-relaxing elbow reflexes. Thyroid function tests show an elevated TSH and low serum T$_4$ level.

Which of these medications might be contributing to her symptoms?

A Amiodarone
B Fluoxetine
C Lisinopril
D Prednisolone
E Simvastatin

15. Painful fingers

A 52-year-old woman presents with a 2-year history of painful fingers. In cold weather her fingers turn pale and then through blue to red, at which point she experiences severe pain in the fingers. Over the last few months, she has had some retrosternal pain on eating and experiences some reflux. On examination the fingers appear to be swollen and tense, with some dilated nail-fold capillary loops, and a small, crusted ulcer is present on a fingertip.

What is the most likely diagnosis?

A Dermatomyositis
B Limited cutaneous systemic sclerosis
C Primary Raynaud phenomenon
D Sarcoidosis
E Systemic lupus erythematosus

16. Palpitations

A 26-year-old woman presents to the GP with a history of palpitations. She also feels hot most of the time and has noticed some weight loss. On examination, she has a "startled" look with lid lag and lid retraction. There is a palpable neck lump on examination that moves up on swallowing.

Which of the following investigations will be LEAST appropriate?

A 24-hour electrocardiogram
B Technetium-99 scintigraphy
C Fine-needle aspiration
D Thyroid function tests
E TSH-receptor antibodies

17. Haemoptysis

A 15-year-old boy has recently started coughing up blood. He has had a non-productive cough for about 6 months with intermittent haemoptysis. Otherwise, he is normally fit and well. On examination, finger clubbing is noted. Chest examination reveals basal crepitations with reduced air entry. Pulmonary function tests reveal a raised transfer factor. A blood test shows low haemoglobin, low mean cell volume, low iron and low ferritin. Autoantibody profiling is negative.

What is the most likely diagnosis?

A Goodpasture syndrome
B Idiopathic pulmonary haemosiderosis
C Microscopic polyarteritis
D Systemic lupus erythematosus
E Granulomatosis with polyangiitis (formally known as Wegener granulomatosis)

18. Antibody testing

A 64-year-old woman presents with a 3-week history of progressive painless haematuria, hypertension, breathlessness and haemoptysis. There is no evidence of epistaxis. Her blood pressure is now 190/110 mmHg, and her chest X-ray shows haemorrhagic pulmonary infiltrates in the lower zones. Her bloods reveal a creatinine level of 340 μmol/L and a raised C-reactive protein.

Which of the following antibody tests would confirm the likely diagnosis?

A Anti–double-stranded DNA antibodies (anti-dsDNA)
B Anti–glomerular basement membrane antibodies (anti-GBM)
C Anti-ribonucleoprotein antibodies (anti-RNP)
D Cytoplasmic antineutrophil cytoplasm antibodies (cANCA)
E Perinuclear antineutrophil cytoplasm antibodies (pANCA)

19. Management of shortness of breath

A 60-year-old man presents to the emergency department with progressive breathlessness on exertion. He has a past medical history of hypertension, diabetes mellitus and chronic obstructive pulmonary disease. He has also complained of weight loss for the past 6 months. On examination, he was alert with a respiratory rate of 25/min and an oxygen saturation reading of 86% in air. He has distended neck veins, facial oedema and bilateral arm swelling.

Which of the following management options is NOT appropriate initially?

A Consider intravenous dexamethasone and radiotherapy
B Consider intubation if in respiratory compromise
C Consider percutaneous endovascular stenting
D Give oxygen to maintain saturation at 88–92%
E Request a chest X-ray

20. Atrial fibrillation

Which of the following is NOT a cause of atrial fibrillation?

A Abdominal aortic aneurysm
B Acute infection
C Binge drinking
D Hypertension
E Idiopathic

21. Blood groups

Which of the following is the universal recipient in blood transfusion?

A A+
B AB–
C AB+
D B–
E O

22. Generalised weakness

A 43-year-old woman presents to the GP with generalised weakness. She notices that she has been gaining weight for the past 3 months despite a normal diet. She has a past medical history of asthma, which is poorly controlled, and she was admitted to the hospital twice last year due to exacerbations. On examination, her blood pressure is 160/90 mmHg. She has bruises on both shins, with wasting and weakness of her proximal thigh muscles.

Which of the following is the most likely diagnosis?

A Addison's disease
B Cushing's syndrome
C Hypothyroidism
D Hyperthyroidism
E Hypercalcaemia

23. Investigation of jaundice

A 25-year-old female student, who is normally fit and well, presents to the emergency department 3 weeks before her final exams. She is drowsy and confused. On examination, she has a hepatic flap and is jaundiced. There is also tender hepatomegaly.

Which of the following is a pertinent first-line investigation?

A Ferritin levels
B Gamma-glutamyl transferase (GGT)
C Hepatitis screen
D Lumbar puncture
E Paracetamol levels

24. Management of skin conditions

An 83-year-old woman who lives in a care home presents with a 2-week history of itching. A few of the other residents have since complained of similar symptoms. You suspect scabies.

Which of the following statements about scabies is FALSE?

A All clothes, bedsheets and any upholstery contacted by the patient should be washed thoroughly

B Burrows are often in web spaces of the digits, wrists, elbows and male genitals

C Diagnosis is by examining scraped-off burrows under a microscope

D Treatment is application of topical malathion or permethrin

E Treatment with topical agents can be one-off or can ideally be repeated 7 days later

25. Investigation of muscle weakness

A 35-year-old woman presents with a history of weakness and paraesthesia for 2 weeks. It started with some unusual sensations in her feet and hands, then some days later she noticed her feet were dragging as she walked. Then over the next week she became unable to get out of her chair and developed arm weakness. She says she had some diarrhoea and abdominal cramps around 4 weeks ago. On examination there is weakness throughout the legs and arms in a patchy distribution varying between grades 2 and 4, reflexes are diminished throughout and there is reduced sensation in the feet up to mid-shin level.

Which of the following investigation findings is suggestive of the likely diagnosis?

A Multifocal decreased motor conduction block only

B Multifocal decreased motor conduction speed with and without conduction block

C Oligoclonal bands on lumbar puncture

D Positive antiviral or antibacterial antibodies to *Campylobacter*

E Raised lymphocytes on lumbar puncture

26. Hepatitis serology

A 45-year-old woman presents with malaise, joint pains and jaundice. A hepatitis screen is sent and returns with the following results:

Hepatitis B surface antigen (HBsAg) – POSITIVE
Hepatitis B "e" antigen (HBeAg) – POSITIVE
Hepatitis B core antibody (HBcAb) – POSITIVE

Which of the following is the most likely diagnosis?

A Acute hepatitis B infection

B Chronic hepatitis B infection

C Hepatitis B immunity following previous infection

D Hepatitis B immunity following previous vaccination

E No hepatitis B infection

27. Lumbar puncture

A lumbar puncture in a patient with headache shows the following results:

Cells	460/mm^3 (normal range <4/mm^3)
Predominant cell type	Lymphocytes
Glucose	1.3 mmol/L (normal range 2–9 mmol/L)
Protein	1200 mg/L (normal range 200–400 mg/L)

India ink staining after the culture is negative.

Which one of the following are these findings consistent with?

A Bacterial meningitis
B Cryptococcal meningitis
C Malignant meningitis
D Tubercular meningitis
E Viral meningitis

28. Management of hyperkalaemia

Which of the following medications used in the management of severe hyperkalaemia does not actually lower serum potassium, but rather is cardioprotective by acting as a membrane stabiliser?

A Calcium gluconate
B Calcium Resonium
C Dextrose 50% with Actrapid insulin
D Furosemide
E Salbutamol

29. Management of hypertension

A 60-year-old man with known type 1 diabetes mellitus for the past 20 years has come to his GP for his annual diabetic check. His blood pressure is 160/90 mmHg today. He is found to have a urinary albumin/creatinine ratio (ACR) of >2.5 mg/mmol, suggestive of microalbuminuria.

Which of the following drugs is proven to reduce microalbuminuria?

A ACE inhibitors
B Alpha-blockers
C Beta-blockers
D Calcium channel blockers
E Thiazide

30. Malabsorption

An 18-year-old female is newly diagnosed with coeliac disease following a prolonged history of diarrhoea, malaise and weight loss.

Which of the following is the most suitable initial management?

A Exclusion of gluten from the diet
B Exclusion of lactose from the diet
C Immunosuppressive agents
D Non-steroidal anti-inflammatories
E Stool-forming drugs such as loperamide

31. Brain tumours

Which of the following patients is most likely to have a cerebellopontine angle tumour?

A A 30-year-old woman with unilateral lower motor neurone facial weakness progressing over days and covered in café-au-lait spots
B A 40-year-old woman with insidious-onset unilateral deafness on Weber's testing sound is louder ipsilaterally
C A 50-year-old man with bilateral facial weakness, nasal voice and swallowing difficulty progressing over 3 months
D A 50-year-old woman with insidious-onset unilateral deafness on Weber's testing sound is louder contralaterally and with some ipsilateral reduced facial sensation
E A 65-year-old man with insidious-onset mild bilateral sensorineural deafness and no other neurological abnormality

32. Chest injury

An 85-year-old retired soldier defends a young woman from being mugged, only to find himself stabbed in the left side of the chest.

On arrival at the emergency department, which of the following features would be most relevant?

A Beck's triad
B Kussmaul breathing
C Kussmaul's sign
D Virchow's triad
E Witnessed Stokes–Adams attack

33. Complications of hepatitis infection

A 68-year-old man with chronic hepatitis B virus infection presents with a 1-month history of weight loss, malaise and right upper quadrant discomfort. On examination he has mild ascites and appears cachectic.

What is the most likely diagnosis?

A Cholangiocarcinoma
B Cirrhosis of the liver
C Hepatocellular carcinoma
D Reactivation of hepatitis B
E Right-heart failure

34. Conn's syndrome

You have been asked to explain the causes of hypertension to a patient recently diagnosed with Conn's syndrome.

Which of the following is an incorrect statement that should NOT feature in your explanation?

A Angiotensin I is converted to angiotensin II mainly in the lungs
B Angiotensin II causes blood pressure to rise but will be low in this patient
C Conn's syndrome causes excess aldosterone, the vasoconstriction from which leads to hypertension
D Hypertensive patients are often vulnerable to hypokalaemia as a side effect of their medication
E The patient is vulnerable to hypokalaemia, as they are excreting too much in their urine

35. Dysphagia

An 88-year-old man presents with a month-long history of difficulty swallowing solids. He has noticed his clothes are looser on him now, and he has a significant smoking history.

What is the most likely diagnosis?

A Achalasia
B Lung carcinoma
C Motor neurone disease

D Oesophageal *Candida*
E Oesophageal carcinoma

36. Diagnosis of chest infection

A 71-year-old woman is admitted with 5 days of cough productive of purulent sputum and fevers, which has not improved with oral antibiotics prescribed by the GP. She is now confused and dehydrated with some renal impairment evident from the bloods (urea 9 mmol/L, creatinine 140 μmol/L). Chest X-ray now shows bilateral consolidation.

Urinary antigen testing should be done looking for which causative pathogen?

A *Escherichia coli*
B *Haemophilus influenza*
C *Legionella* spp.

D *Mycoplasma pneumoniae*
E Viruses

37. Diagnosis of cough

A 40-year-old man presents to the GP with an intermittent dry cough (usually nocturnal) over the last 2 months, which has become worse over the past few weeks. Besides that, he also finds himself easily becoming short of breath when he exercises. The cough is dry and non-productive. He does not produce any blood-tinged sputum. He has not lost weight, never smoked and has no other significant past medical history.

What is the most likely diagnosis?

A Asthma
B Chronic obstructive pulmonary disease
C Interstitial pulmonary fibrosis
D Lung cancer
E Pneumonia

38. Diagnosis of Cushing's syndrome

A 40-year-old woman presents to the GP with generalised weakness and weight loss. She noticed that she had become more tanned despite not travelling abroad. On examination, there were bruises on both of her shins. A provisional diagnosis of Cushing's syndrome is made.

Which of the following test is NOT helpful in this case?

A 48-hour high-dose dexamethasone suppression test
B Computed tomography (CT) of the adrenals
C CT of the chest
D Overnight low-dose dexamethasone suppression test
E Plasma ACTH

39. Diagnosis of neurological dysfunction

A 55-year-old man presents with 6 months of progressive weakness in his arms and legs. On further questioning he reveals that he has choked quite a few times recently on swallowing liquids. He is a smoker but has no significant past medical history. He is British and has not travelled widely. On examination of the cranial nerves, his palate does not rise much on the left on saying "aah" and does not rise on the right at all. On examination of his arms, there is wasting of the dorsal interosseous muscles and fasciculations in the right forearm and left deltoid, there is diffuse weakness (grade 4), the reflexes are present or brisk and there is no sensory deficit. On examination of the legs, fasciculations are seen in the thighs, some proximal weakness on the left and brisk knee jerks and upgoing plantar reflexes. Again there is no sensory deficit.

Which of the following diagnoses is most likely?

A Cervical spondylosis
B HIV-related motor neurone disease–like syndrome
C Motor neurone disease
D Multiple sclerosis
E Syringomyelia and syringobulbia

40. Diagnosis of rheumatoid arthritis

A 43-year-old woman presents with a history of 5 months of symmetrical hand pain and swelling with morning stiffness. You suspect rheumatoid arthritis.

Which of the following tests is the most sensitive and specific for rheumatoid arthritis?

A ANCA
B Anti-CCP antibodies
C Anti-centromere antibodies
D Rheumatoid factor
E Soft tissue swelling and bony erosions on X-ray of the hands

41. Diagnosis of skin lesions

A 55-year-old woman presents with a 4-month history of an erythematous rash over her cheeks, nose and forehead. There appear to be multiple small papules and a few pustules on a background of erythematous skin.

What is the most likely diagnosis?

A Acne vulgaris
B Dermatomyositis
C Eczema
D Rosacea
E Systemic lupus erythematosus

42. Electrocardiogram

You are covering the wards overnight. You are bleeped by the critical care ward. An experienced nurse informs you that a recent admission, an 83-year-old woman, has second-degree heart block. You ask her to fax the ECG to you, as you are busy.

What is meant by second-degree heart block?

A A bradycardic QRS complex is dissociated from the P-wave
B Occasional P-waves are failing to conduct through and trigger QRS complexes
C There is a prolonged P-R interval
D There is ST-segment elevation throughout the chest leads
E The QRS complexes are irregularly irregular

43. Emergency management

A 32-year-old man is brought to the emergency department whilst fitting. His airway has been secured using a Guedel airway. He has oxygen saturations above 96% on 15 L of oxygen and a capillary refill time of 2 seconds. Intravenous access has been gained.

Which of the following is the most appropriate next step?

A Jaw thrust
B Intravenous benzylpenicillin
C Intravenous lorazepam
D Intravenous phenytoin
E Rectal diazepam

44. Supraventricular tachycardia

A pleasantly confused 92-year-old woman with a history of cardiac disease is an inpatient on your ward. You are called by a nurse, as her observations are peculiar and she is not feeling well. Her heart rate is 150 bpm and her blood pressure 110/60 mmHg. You inspect her electrocardiogram (ECG) and diagnose a supraventricular tachycardia.

What would be the sensible next step?

A Administer adenosine
B Administer digoxin
C Book an echocardiogram for tomorrow
D Defibrillate
E Print off the ECG and put it in the notes – no further action is required

45. Syndrome of inappropriate ADH secretion

A 68-year-old man presents to hospital with a 2-week history of confusion, and he is found to have a pneumonia, for which he is treated. You note his plasma sodium is 119 mmol/L.

Which of the following investigation findings is consistent with a diagnosis of syndrome of inappropriate antidiuretic hormone secretion (SIADH)?

(Normal values: urine osmolality 50–1200 mOsm/kg, plasma osmolality 280–300 mOsm/kg)

A Urine osmolality 45 mOsm/kg, plasma osmolality 250 mOsm/kg
B Urine osmolality 45 mOsm/kg, plasma osmolality 290 mOsm/kg
C Urine osmolality 45 mOsm/kg, plasma osmolality 305 mOsm/kg
D Urine osmolality 800 mOsm/kg, plasma osmolality 250 mOsm/kg
E Urine osmolality 800 mOsm/kg, plasma osmolality 305 mOsm/kg

46. Systemic lupus erythematosus

A 26-year-old woman presents to the GP with right-sided pleuritic chest pain and increasing exertional dyspnoea that has lasted for about 2 weeks. She also complains of fatigue, malaise, hair loss and arthralgia that has lasted for 3 months. On examination, she has a rash over her cheeks, and auscultation of the chest reveals a friction rub and dullness to percussion over the right lower zone. Autoantibody blood tests demonstrate a profile consistent with systemic lupus erythematosus (SLE).

What is the most likely pulmonary manifestation of SLE in this case?

A Acute pleuritis
B Acute pneumonitis
C Interstitial lung disease
D Pneumonia
E Pulmonary haemorrhage

47. Urinary frequency

A 48-year-old man presents to the emergency department in a reduced state of consciousness. He was brought in by his son who says he has been more confused over the past few days. A collateral history suggests 2 weeks of polyuria and polydipsia. There was no history of head injury, trauma or ingestion of illegal drugs. He has no other significant past medical history. He has a 21-unit/week alcohol history. On examination, he is unresponsive to pain. The liver edge is felt on abdominal examination. His blood tests show the following:

Na^+	168 mmol/L
K^+	3.8 mmol/L
Glucose	68 mmol/L
Serum osmolality	350 mmol/kg
Urea	14.3 mmol/L
Creatinine	203 μmol/L

A urine dipstick test revealed glycosuria but no ketones.

What is the most likely differential diagnosis?

A Diabetic ketoacidosis
B Encephalitis
C Hepatic encephalopathy
D Hyperosmolar hyperglycaemic state (HHS)
E Uraemia

48. Wilson's disease

A 24-year-old man diagnosed with Wilson's disease was started on penicillamine. He calls his GP 1 month later to report that he has a temperature and a sore throat and has noticed marked bruising in the last week.

What advice should the GP give at this time?

A Advise the patient this is likely to be flu
B Ask the patient to come in for an urgent blood test
C Ask the patient to take some paracetamol and book an appointment the following week
D Increase the dose of penicillamine
E Reconsider the diagnosis of Wilson's disease

49. X-ray changes in osteoarthritis

Which of the following radiographic changes is NOT consistent with a diagnosis of osteoarthritis?

A Loss of joint space
B Osteophytes
C Punched-out periarticular erosions
D Subarticular sclerosis
E Subchondral cysts

50. Traveller's diarrhoea

A 22-year-old male medical student returns from travelling across Southeast Asia with a 48-hour history of watery diarrhoea and abdominal pain. He is otherwise well in himself.

What is the most common organism for a short history of traveller's diarrhoea?

A Amoebic dysentery
B *Escherichia coli*
C *Listeria*
D Malaria
E *Salmonella*

Practice paper 6: Answers

1. Amenorrhoea

B. Karyotype analysis

This patient has Turner's syndrome, characterised by short stature and primary amenorrhoea due to loss of part or all of an X chromosome. Other features include a broad square-shaped chest, widely spaced nipples, a webbed neck, a high palate and short fourth metacarpals. Most affected females have no pubertal development and primary amenorrhoea. There are, however, some who develop normally and have secondary amenorrhoea. Patients with Turner's syndrome may have other complications such as renal anomalies (horseshoe kidneys); cardiovascular disease/abnormalities (coarctation of the aorta, aortic valvular disease, aortic dissection, hypertension); osteoporosis; ocular abnormalities; and hypothyroidism. Karyotype analysis is used to analyse the chromosomal composition of the individual, which would reveal an abnormal or missing X chromosome in these females (45, XO).

Henry Turner, American endocrinologist (1892-1970)

2. Myasthenia gravis

D. Rimmed vacuoles on muscle biopsy

In the Tensilon test, edrophonium (a very short-acting cholinesterase inhibitor) is administered; if positive, the weakness markedly improves for around 2–4 minutes. Positivity suggests myasthenia gravis, although it can be positive in the Lambert–Eaton myasthenic syndrome. Electromyography commonly reveals that with repeated stimulation of the motor nerve fibres, the amplitude of the muscle action potentials reduce – a "decrementing response". This seems to represent the classic fatigability of the weakness in myasthenia gravis. A more sensitive test is looking at "jitter" – the variability of action potential time interval between two different single-motor fibres of the same motor unit. Acetylcholine receptor antibodies are found in at least 90% of patients and, with increased sensitivity of new assays, it is thought that 96% actually may be positive. In many negative patients, antibodies to muscle-specific kinase (MuSK) are found. In any new patient, a

DOI: 10.1201/9781003648222-12

CT of the chest should be carried out to look for thymoma, found in 10% of patients. Hyperplasia is found in a further 70% of patients. Rimmed vacuoles are in fact a hallmark of the rare inclusion body myositis, which can present with distal myopathy. Muscle biopsy may reveal muscle fibre atrophy and can show small necrotic foci of damage or diffuse necrosis and inflammation, depending on disease severity.

3. Hyperkalaemia

B. Deepening Q-waves

A potassium level >7 mmol/L is a medical emergency and can be asymptomatic until arrest. ECG monitoring should be set up to look for early changes, and the ECG compared to a previous ECG from when the patient was stable (if available). The T-waves tent because potassium influx into cells drives repolarisation, and ventricular repolarisation is represented by the T-wave – the higher extracellular potassium concentrations lead to a larger magnitude of depolarisation. The P-waves flatten (although this may be subtle) and the QRS complexes broaden. A finding of any of these changes should increase urgency of treatment, during which ECG monitoring should continue. The changes progress to reveal a "sine wave" pattern, and ventricular fibrillation can ensue if appropriate treatment is not instituted (usually when K^+ >9). Deepening Q-waves would be associated with evolution of an ST-elevation myocardial infarction, with the initial ST elevation decreasing and the Q-waves deepening hours to days after the infarct.

4. Myocardial infarction

D. Nuclear studies of the myocardium

Single-photon emission computed tomography (SPECT) is a nuclear medicine scan involving gamma rays. It relies on the injection of a gamma-emitting radioisotope (a radionuclide), which is taken up by healthy myocardium. A sequence of images of the myocardium is then taken to highlight any perfusion deficiencies and ventricular dysfunction. Infarcted myocardium will be clearly displayed. Troponin tests can also be positive in heart failure and are therefore not sensitive enough in this context.

5. Pruritus

A. Electrolytes

A full blood count can reveal anaemia (which may be due to iron deficiency), polycythaemia, lymphoma or leukaemia, all of which can cause pruritus. Polycythaemia characteristically causes itching upon bathing. Iron studies can reveal a low ferritin and thus iron deficiency, which can cause pruritus. However, a cause should be sought, including gastrointestinal bleeding, menorrhagia and diet. Hyperthyroidism and hypothyroidism can both cause itching. Chronic renal failure can cause an intractable pruritus, which unfortunately is often not relieved by dialysis; thus, measuring urea is useful. Electrolyte abnormalities do not cause pruritus. A full and thorough history and examination can guide towards a potential diagnosis; however, subclinical disease may be evident on blood tests – hence the pruritus screen. Other indicated blood tests include liver function tests (bile salt deposited in the skin can cause itching). If all tests are negative, psychological factors can often play a part, with anxiety being the most common cause. The tests can be repeated at intervals if patients re-present and/or psychological factors seem unlikely.

Pruritus, from Latin *prurire* = to itch

6. Seizures

C. Shooting/electric shock–like pains in the limbs

Complex partial seizures usually originate in the temporal lobe and can affect various components of the limbic system, including the hippocampus. The limbic system has various functions including memory, emotion, taste and smell and consciousness. Therefore, complex partial seizures present with episodes of clouding of consciousness combined with various symptoms that may include visceral symptoms (fullness, choking, nausea, tachycardia, taste and smell hallucinations); memory disturbance (déjà-vu, jamais-vu, derealisation, flashbacks, formed auditory or visual hallucinations); motor disturbances of a semi-purposeful nature; or intense paroxysmal mood disturbance. Shooting pains into the limbs, depending on the distribution, sound typical of a radiculopathy, and "electric shock" sensations sound like "Lhermitte's sign", a sign in multiple sclerosis with cervical posterior column involvement, whereby sudden neck flexion causes electric shock–like sensations in the limbs. Focal somatosensory or pain information is not processed in the temporal lobe or limbic system anyhow and so is unlikely to be caused by complex partial seizures.

Jean Lhermitte, French neurologist (1877-1959)

7. Spinal cord compression

D. T10

Complete involvement of the legs in either sensory or motor modality indicates that the lesion is higher than L1. The arms are normal, so the lesion is lower than T1. Getting the answer, then, depends on knowledge of anatomical landmarks of spinal sensory levels. T4 is the level of the nipples, which does not help us narrow the answer down. T10 is the level of the bellybutton, and thus T10 is the answer we are looking for. The cause of greatest concern is metastases – magnetic resonance imaging (MRI) of the spine may discover this or another cause and gauge the extent of spinal compression if that is indeed the cause.

8. Sepsis

C. Neutrophils <0.5 × 10⁹/L

The combination of a raised temperature and low neutrophils (<1 or <0.5 × 10^9/L; the precise value varies according to local policy) is described as neutropenic sepsis. Patients receiving chemotherapy often drop their neutrophil count due to bone marrow suppression, and the relative paucity of neutrophils means that the host defence against bacteria is severely compromised. These patients can die rapidly despite not being clinically drastically unwell. It is essential to start broad-spectrum intravenous antibiotics as soon as possible. Blood cultures can be taken afterwards if necessary.

9. Radiographic changes in ankylosing spondylitis

D. Sacroiliitis

Fusion of the sacroiliac joints and fusion of the lumbar vertebra (giving the "bamboo spine") happen only after prolonged persistent inflammation leads to calcification of the ligaments. Osteophytes are seen in osteoarthritis and in degenerative spinal disease (spondylosis). Syndesmophytes are bony spurs caused by persistent inflammation that are more vertically oriented than osteophytes and represent an earlier stage of disease than bamboo spine. The earliest radiographic change in ankylosing spondylitis is sacroiliitis.

10. Management of toxicity

D. Give intravenous naloxone

Opiate toxicity in patients causes reduced consciousness, respiratory depression, pinpoint pupils and hypotension. In the case of reduced conscious level or respiratory depression, aliquots of 0.4–2.0 mg intravenous naloxone should be given, and the dose might need repeating if there is inadequate response after 2 minutes. A naloxone infusion might be needed in the case of known severe opiate toxicity (e.g. long-acting opiates such as sustained release morphine sulphate or methadone). *N*-acetylcysteine is used in paracetamol overdose. Flumazenil is used in benzodiazepine overdose. Sodium bicarbonate is used in salicylate poisoning. Torsades de pointes induced by antidepressant overdose (e.g. selective serotonin reuptake inhibitors) is treated with intravenous magnesium sulphate.

11. Squamous cell carcinoma

A. Curettage is the first line of management

Curettage is unlikely to remove the whole tumour and will lead to delay in clearance of the malignant cells. Primary excision should be the first line of management. Mohs micrographic surgery, whereby excised samples are examined under the microscope at the time of excision and then further tissue resected until the margins are clear, can be used for high-risk recurrent lesions. Radiotherapy can be used where excision is not possible, and chemotherapy can be used in metastatic disease. Sun exposure is indeed a risk factor for squamous cell carcinoma, which tends to present as ill-defined, keratotic, ulcerating lesions. The lesions are more common in kidney transplant patients because of the long-term immunosuppression – another risk factor. Unlike basal cell carcinomas, squamous cell carcinomas can indeed metastasise, usually to lymph nodes, so if histopathology confirms a squamous cell carcinoma, annual follow-up for 5 years to exclude lymphadenopathy or recurrent malignancy is recommended.

Frederic Edward Mohs, American surgeon (1910-2002)

12. Management of urinary tract infection

B. Leukocyte esterase negative, nitrites negative, but >10^5/mL Gram-negative rods on microscopy

The presence of either leukocyte esterase or nitrites may be a common finding in the urine dip of a pregnant woman. The prompt recognition of an infection is crucial to minimise the risk of ascending infection and renal damage. However, treatment should only be started in asymptomatic patients in the presence of a urine culture confirming bacteriuria. Possible antibiotics that are not contraindicated in pregnancy include nitrofurantoin, amoxicillin and cephalexin.

13. Side effects of anti-tuberculous medication

A. Ethambutol

Ethambutol can cause optic neuritis, which initially affects the myelinated nerves supplying the cones in the fovea. Thus, loss of colour vision and visual acuity can be the earliest presenting features. If picked up early, stopping the ethambutol can lead to reversal of the process and the vision saved. Isoniazid, pyrazinamide and rifampicin, along with the ethambutol, comprise standard quadruple therapy, which will be given for the first 2 months in new tuberculosis, before continuing the isoniazid and rifampicin for a further 4 months. All three can cause hepatitis. Isoniazid can cause peripheral neuropathy via a vitamin B_6 deficiency, so prophylactic pyridoxine is prescribed. Rifampicin is an enzyme inducer and can interact with many other medications, notably the oral contraceptive pill. It can also turn body secretions orange. Streptomycin can be used in place of ethambutol or in combination with all four in resistant tuberculosis.

14. Hypothyroidism

A. Amiodarone

Amiodarone has a chemical structure that is analogous to thyroxine and contains large amounts of iodine. Amiodarone has a cytotoxic effect on thyroid follicular cells and inhibits conversion of T_4 to T_3. As a result, either hypothyroidism (Wolff–Chaikoff effect) or hyperthyroidism (Jod–Basedow effect) may occur. Thyroid function tests should be done before commencement of amiodarone, and thyroid-stimulating hormone should be measured every 6 months whilst the patient is on treatment.

15. Painful fingers

B. Limited cutaneous systemic sclerosis

Systemic sclerosis is a connective tissue disorder characterised by thickening and fibrosis of the skin (scleroderma) with involvement of internal organs. There are two forms: (1) a limited cutaneous type (60%) and (2) a diffuse cutaneous type (40%). Limited cutaneous scleroderma is limited to the distal limbs (i.e. distal to the elbows and knees). Other features include a beaked nose and small, furrowed mouth (microstoma). Limited cutaneous scleroderma also encompasses CREST syndrome, which is characterised by calcinosis, Raynaud phenomenon, oesophageal dysmotility, sclerodactyly and telangiectasia. Calcinosis is the formation of calcium deposits in the soft tissues, often seen on the pulps of the fingers. Raynaud's phenomenon is an idiopathic condition with episodic digital vasospasm precipitated by a cold environment; consequently, the affected fingers or toes become white and may be painful. Oesophageal dysmotility may manifest as dysphagia and reflux. Sclerodactyly describes the presence of tight, shiny skin over the fingers, producing a fixed flexion deformity. In limited cutaneous scleroderma the anti-centromere antibody is characteristically positive. Pulmonary hypertension is a common internal manifestation.

Diffuse cutaneous scleroderma can involve the skin of the entire body. Patients are characteristically positive for the anti–SCL-70 antibody (also known as anti-topoisomerase II). In this form of disease, patients are particularly at risk of a "renal crisis" – a life-threatening malignant hypertension with rapid renal impairment. By contrast, pulmonary hypertension is less common. Diffuse cutaneous systemic sclerosis has a worse prognosis than limited cutaneous disease. The treatment of systemic sclerosis is with steroids and immunosuppressant agents. Penicillamine slows skin disease (steroids do not help the skin). Lung fibrosis is the main cause of death, followed by renal disease.

Scleroderma can occur without internal organ disease (localised scleroderma). If this occurs in plaques, it is known as morphea; if it occurs in lines, it is termed *en coup de sabre.* "Scleroderma sine scleroderma" is the name given to patients who have typical vascular or internal organ features of systemic sclerosis but without the cutaneous sclerosis.

Dermatomyositis, another connective tissue disease, can feature dilated nail-fold capillary loops, but this presentation is not of dermatomyositis – we would expect a proximal muscle weakness and pain with possible skin manifestations, including heliotropic rash around the eyes and Gottron's papules on the dorsum of the hands.

Morphea, from Greek *morpha* = shape

En coup de sabre, from French = cut of the sword

Scleroderma, from Latin *skleros* = hard + *dermis* = skin

Maurice Raynaud, French physician (1834–1881)

16. Palpitations

A. 24-hour electrocardiogram

The clinical features of this patient suggest thyrotoxicosis. Patients with primary thyrotoxicosis would have raised T_3 and T_4 with an undetectable thyroid-stimulating hormone (TSH). TSH receptor antibody levels are raised in Graves' disease. An ECG may demonstrate atrial fibrillation. The technetium-99 scintigraphy scan would demonstrate the distribution of the uptake of the isotope: (1) in Graves' disease there is a diffuse uptake of isotope, (2) in multinodular goitre there is low patchy uptake within the nodules, and (3) in toxic adenomas there is lack of uptake of isotope by the normal dormant gland. Fine-needle aspiration confirms the cytology of the thyroid nodule. A 24-hour electrocardiogram (ECG) may demonstrate atrial fibrillation, but it is not essential in the diagnosis of thyrotoxicosis.

17. Haemoptysis

B. Idiopathic pulmonary haemosiderosis

Idiopathic pulmonary haemosiderosis is a rare condition with unknown aetiology that is characterised by recurrent episodes of alveolar haemorrhage and haemoptysis (in the absence of renal disease) and leads to iron-deficiency anaemia. Most patients present in childhood, with 85% of cases having an onset of symptoms before 16 years of age. The aetiology is thought to be multifactorial with possible associations with toxin exposure and an autoimmune mechanism. The alveolar and interstitial spaces are filled with haemosiderin-laden macrophages with variable extent of interstitial fibrosis and degeneration of alveolar, interstitial and vascular elastic fibres. The clinical course of this condition ranges from continuous low-level bleeding to massive pulmonary haemorrhage. Continuous pulmonary haemorrhage leads to the chronic non-productive cough with haemoptysis, malaise, lethargy and failure to thrive in children. Causes of diffuse alveolar haemorrhage include systemic lupus erythematosus (SLE), eosinophilic granulomatosis with polyangiitis (formally known as Churg–Strauss syndrome) and granulomatosis with polyangiitis (formally known as Wegener granulomatosis). Chronic bleeding leads to iron-deficiency anaemia, chronic disabling dyspnoea, pulmonary fibrosis and cor pulmonale.

18. Antibody testing

B. Anti–glomerular basement membrane antibodies (anti-GBM)

This patient has Goodpasture's syndrome, which is a rare condition in which autoantibodies are formed against the glomerular basement membrane and the alveolar membrane. The antibodies trigger a type 2 hypersensitivity reaction that causes renal failure, pulmonary haemorrhage and haemoptysis. The condition is usually diagnosed by the detection of anti-GBM in the serum and via renal biopsy. The biopsy often shows focal or diffuse crescentic glomerulonephritis. Immunofluorescence may demonstrate linear deposition of IgG antibodies and complement (C3) on the glomerular basement membrane. Goodpasture's syndrome is usually treated aggressively with plasmapheresis, corticosteroids and immunosuppression.

Anti-dsDNA antibodies are found in systemic lupus erythematosus (SLE), and whilst only 60% are sensitive (compared to >95% with antinuclear antibodies [ANAs]), it is far more specific. Lupus can cause renal disease, typically with proteinuria and/or casts rather than haematuria, and can affect the lungs through pleuritis or pleural effusions, but it does not cause haemoptysis. Anti-ribonucleoprotein antibodies are specific for mixed connective tissue disease, which would be unlikely to give the present clinical picture. Cytoplasmic antineutrophil cytoplasm antibodies (cANCAs) are most associated with Wegener's granulomatosis, which could cause a similar picture with renal impairment of a nephritic type and haemoptysis. It is also sometimes found in Churg–Strauss syndrome, microscopic polyangiitis and polyarteritis nodosa. Perinuclear antineutrophil cytoplasmic antibodies (pANCAs) are found most often in microscopic polyangiitis and can actually sometimes be positive in Goodpasture's syndrome.

Ernest William Goodpasture, American pathologist (1886-1960)

19. Management of shortness of breath

A. Consider intravenous dexamethasone and radiotherapy

Superior vena cava syndrome is a clinical condition that occurs due to obstruction of the superior vena cava. The most common aetiology is malignancy (65% of cases), and this is followed by benign causes, which include iatrogenic causes (e.g. central venous catheters, pacemaker), mediastinal fibrosis caused by radiotherapy or infections, collagen-vascular diseases (e.g. sarcoidosis or Behçet syndrome) and, rarely, mediastinal haematoma, substernal goitre and aortic arch aneurysm. The most common malignant cause is lung cancer, followed by lymphoma, metastatic breast cancer and metastatic colon cancer. Patients present with dyspnoea, cough, facial plethora, oedema of the upper extremities and distended neck veins and chest veins, and in severe cases, they have stridor related to laryngeal oedema or direct compression. Oxygen should be provided to correct hypoxaemia. A chest X-ray might reveal a widened mediastinum and a mass lesion. Airway management is important, as the patient might have upper airway obstruction due to severe oedema, and intubation should be considered in these cases. Corticosteroids and radiation therapy or percutaneous stenting is considered for the relief of obstructive symptoms. Urgent combination therapy with radiotherapy and corticosteroids are only used in life-threatening situations, as they might cause interference with subsequent histopathological diagnosis in patients who do not have histopathological evidence of malignancy.

20. Atrial fibrillation

A. Abdominal aortic aneurysm

Atrial fibrillation commonly presents with either missing P-waves on the electrocardiogram (ECG) or, as beautifully described in 1876 by Carl Nothnagel:

> In this form of arrhythmia the heartbeats follow each other in complete irregularity. At the same time, the height and tension of the individual pulse waves are continuously changing.

Because the atria are not efficiently contracting, blood can clot within the left atrium and result in embolisation.

Causes of atrial fibrillation can be remembered using **Dehydrated PIRATES**:

- **Dehydration**
- **P**ulmonary disease, e.g. pulmonary embolism
- **I**schaemia (hypertension, ischaemic heart disease, heart failure)
- **R**heumatic heart disease

- Anaemia, atrial myxoma
- Thyrotoxicosis
- Ethanol abuse
- Sepsis

21. Blood groups

C. AB+

Blood groups A and B represent antigens present on the surface of the red blood cell. Blood type O indicates the absence of these antigens. Through our diets we are exposed to all antigens and therefore build up antibodies to any foreign antigens. For example a person with blood type O, and therefore no native antigen chains (universal donor if Rhesus negative), will have antibodies to both A and B chains. However, a person who has both AB on their own cells will not produce antibodies and can therefore receive all blood (universal recipient if Rhesus positive). Although the ABO compatibility is the most important blood typing system, more than 30 other blood typing systems are known. Rhesus compatibility is demonstrated by the plus or minus symbol.

22. Generalised weakness

B. Cushing's syndrome

Cushing's syndrome is caused by the excessive activation of glucocorticoid receptors. The most common cause is iatrogenic secondary to prolonged use of synthetic glucocorticoids such as prednisolone. The degree to which symptoms manifest is dependent on the degree of cortisol excess. Patients will complain of abnormal centripetal weight gain ("orange on a stick" appearance), acne, striae, abnormal bruising and weakness involving their proximal muscles. They may be found to be hyperglycaemic, hypertensive and are prone to infections with poor wound healing. A history of poor asthma control suggests that patient is on long-term steroid therapy, which is the main cause of her Cushing's syndrome.

Harvey Williams Cushing, American neurosurgeon (1869-1939)

23. Investigation of jaundice

E. Paracetamol levels

This patient is most likely to have taken an overdose of paracetamol, which has resulted in the features of acute liver failure demonstrated earlier. Alcohol can cause a similar picture in the long term but not in the acute setting. Paracetamol overdose in the first 24 hours presents with non-specific symptoms of nausea and vomiting. Hepatic necrosis begins 24 hours after the overdose with the classic signs of acute liver failure. Initial investigations need to include liver function tests (LFTs), paracetamol and salicylate levels, blood glucose (as such patients are prone to hypoglycaemia), urea and electrolytes (think hepatorenal syndrome, although urea is synthesised in the liver and so may not be deranged), clotting and an arterial blood gas looking for lactic acidosis. If patients with a paracetamol overdose present within 1 hour, you can consider giving activated charcoal to prevent absorption. A 4-hour paracetamol level can be used to determine which patients would benefit from *N*-acetylcysteine infusions (paracetamol level at 4 hours is charted on the Rumack–Matthew normogram). Maximum protection is gained by giving the antidote within 8 hours of ingestion.

24. Management of skin conditions

A. All clothes, bedsheets and any upholstery contacted by the patient should be washed thoroughly

Scabies is caused by parasitic mites that burrow under the skin and lay their eggs, eventually causing a hypersensitivity reaction that causes the itch. Washing clothes, underwear, nightclothes, bedsheets and towels used in the 3 days prior to diagnosis suffices to cover potential lurking mites that may reinfect the individual after treatment. Burrows, which can often be linear lesions representing the path burrowed by the mite, have a vesicle at the end of the mite and are indeed often found in the web spaces of fingers and toes, as well as hands and feet, wrists and ankles, elbows, nipples and male genitalia. For diagnosis, a burrow (not those on the genitalia) should be scraped off and examined under the microscope directly. A dermatoscope can sometimes visualise the mite in situ in the burrow on the patient. Malathion and permethrin are both valid topical treatments, which should be applied all over. Permethrin can be washed off after 12 hours, malathion after 24 hours. A second application 7 days later is often recommended to sweep up any mites missed by the first treatment.

Scabies, from Latin *scabere* = to itch

25. Investigation of muscle weakness

B. Multifocal decreased motor conduction speed with and without conduction block

Guillain–Barré syndrome (GBS) is the eponym for acute inflammatory postinfectious polyneuropathy. It commonly follows viral infection, e.g. varicella zoster virus, mumps and cytomegalovirus, or bacterial infections such as *Campylobacter* or *Mycoplasma*. However, serology confirming prior infection with one of these organisms does not confirm GBS. Lumbar puncture commonly reveals raised protein, but lymphocytes are not usually raised, and oligoclonal bands would not be expected. The underlying pathology is an autoimmune attack on the myelin in the peripheral nerves, and so slowed motor conduction speed would be expected. If the inflammation is severe, axons can be damaged, giving a conduction block picture. This indicates that a degree of irreversible damage has taken place. There is a 2% mortality rate in GBS, and of those who develop respiratory failure, 20% are left severely disabled. Therapy is with intravenous immunoglobulin if the patient is unable to walk.

Georges Guillain, French neurologist (1876-1961)

Jean Alexandre Barré, French neurologist (1880-1967)

26. Hepatitis serology

A. Acute hepatitis B infection

The immunological tests for hepatitis B can be complicated and confusing; however, they also can be very helpful in determining the current hepatitis status of the patient, as well as their previous exposure. Hepatitis B is a DNA virus that is mainly transmitted via blood products and sexual activity. Certain individuals, such as those who work in healthcare, are required to be vaccinated against hepatitis B. The vaccine contains the hepatitis surface antigen (HBsAg) against which the immune system produces hepatitis B surface antibody (HBsAb). It is HBsAb that is measured after vaccination to evaluate the response to the vaccine. Some individuals have a poor response to the vaccine and require higher doses or booster shots. HBsAb is also found in patients who have had hepatitis in the past. In this situation the patient will also have developed antibodies to the hepatitis B core antigen (HBcAg), which is not present in patients who have been immunised.

Hepatitis B surface antigen (HBsAg) can usually be detected within 4 weeks of infection and is the earliest marker of infection. It is not found in patients vaccinated against hepatitis B. If HBsAg is still detected in the serum 6 months after an acute hepatitis B infection, the patient has become a chronic carrier of the virus. The risk of developing chronic hepatitis B infection is related to age at the time of infection. The majority of infected neonates develop chronic infection, whereas only 5–10% of adults do so.

Hepatitis B "e" antigen (HBeAg) can be present in both acute and chronic hepatitis B and indicates a high level of infectivity. The presence of HBeAg in chronic hepatitis B suggests that the patient is infective and has an aggressive disease requiring treatment. In addition to establishing infectivity, the measurement of HBeAg can be used to assess the efficacy of treatment, with falling levels indicating success. It should be noted that some mutant strains of the hepatitis B virus are found in Asia and the Middle East that do not produce HBeAg. Hepatitis B DNA levels can also be used to assess disease activity, with high levels indicating active disease and infectivity.

Hepatitis B core antibodies (HBcAb) can be present in acute and chronic infection. They are formed against the hepatitis B core antigen (HBcAg), which is found within the liver and therefore cannot be detected using serology. In acute infection it is the second marker to be detected, after HBsAb, and is usually seen after 4 weeks of infection. In chronic disease the presence of high titres of HBcAb, in the absence of HBeAg, indicates low infectivity and disease activity. This serological picture is associated with a better prognosis, with fewer individuals progressing to cirrhosis and hepatocellular carcinoma.

27. Lumbar puncture

D. Tubercular meningitis

The glucose is low, indicating excessive glucose consumption, which rules out viral meningitis. The predominance of lymphocytes suggests a more chronic infection and rules out bacterial meningitis. The negative India ink stain rules out cryptococcal meningitis. Finally, the extremely large number of lymphocytes and amount of protein make tuberculosis more likely than malignant meningitis. Ziehl–Neelsen staining or polymerase chain reaction (PCR) would confirm the diagnosis. However, clinical information, conspicuously absent from this case, would be extremely useful.

28. Management of hyperkalaemia

A. Calcium gluconate

Hyperkalaemia is defined as a serum potassium level of >5 mmol/L, but severe hyperkalaemia is present when serum potassium levels exceed 7 mmol/L and is considered a medical emergency. ECG monitoring should be instituted and intravenous access sought. Calcium gluconate does not lower serum potassium, but 10 ml of 10% calcium gluconate is given as a cardioprotective agent, as it is a cardiac membrane stabiliser and protects against cardiac arrhythmias. This should be given soon, as it can buy time to lower the potassium level. Dextrose (50 ml of 50% solution) with 10 units Actrapid insulin can be given intravenously – insulin drives potassium rapidly into cells, and the dextrose is given with it to avoid hypoglycaemia. Potassium and glucose levels should then be monitored repeatedly. Calcium Resonium, typically given as a 30-mg suppository, soaks up potassium from the bowel wall, and then an enema after 9 hours will actually remove potassium from the body. Calcium Resonium can also be given orally (15 mg TDS) with laxatives to speed transit time. The cause for the high potassium should be sought and reversed where possible. Medications such as beta-blockers, angiotensin-converting enzyme (ACE) inhibitors, potassium-sparing diuretics such as spironolactone and non-steroidal anti-inflammatory drugs (NSAIDs) can contribute and should be stopped.

Hyperglycaemia can be responsible, as can causes of cell lysis such as burns and rhabdomyolysis. Acute or chronic renal failure is often responsible, and if acute renal failure is not reversible by other means, then dialysis will be needed, and this often is the definitive means of reducing the serum potassium. Furosemide is a loop diuretic and causes potassium loss through the kidney, but if the patient is clinically dry or has renal failure, this may be unsafe. Salbutamol nebulisers can be used to drive potassium into cells, but the high doses needed lead to side effects such as tachycardia, anxiety and tremors, which are undesirable in an already unwell patient.

29. Management of hypertension

A. ACE inhibitors

Diabetic nephropathy is among the most common causes of end-stage renal failure in developed countries. Microalbuminuria is an important indicator of risk of developing overt diabetic nephropathy. Blood pressure control is associated with reduction of proteinuria and a reduction in the rate of chronic kidney disease progression. Angiotensin-converting enzyme (ACE) inhibitors dilate the efferent renal arteriole, thus reducing intraglomerular hypertension and proteinuria, regardless of whether blood pressure is elevated or not.

30. Malabsorption

A. Exclusion of gluten from the diet

Coeliac disease causes a gluten-related enteropathy of the small bowel. When the patient consumes gluten-containing foods, a T-cell–mediated autoimmune reaction results in subtotal villous atrophy and crypt hyperplasia of the small bowel mucosa. Specifically, it is gliadin – a constituent of gluten – which causes the immunological response. The result is malabsorption leading to malnutrition, anaemia, steatorrhoea, abdominal pain, bloating and fatigue. Patients are at risk of developing deficiencies in iron, vitamin B_{12}, folate, calcium and vitamin D due to malabsorption. The initial investigation for coeliac disease is the measurement of serum anti-endomyseal or anti-transglutaminase IgA antibodies, which have been shown to have sensitivities and specificities of over 95%. Antibodies to alpha-gliadin and reticulin can also be measured, although they have lower sensitivities and specificities. The gold standard diagnostic technique is duodenal or jejunal biopsy taken during endoscopy. Gluten exclusion can reverse the disease process, and therefore biopsy must occur before exclusion starts. Since this is an invasive and unpleasant procedure, it is usually performed as a second-line investigation in patients with positive serology. If the biopsy suggests coeliac disease, the patient should be placed on a gluten-free diet and re-biopsied at a later date to assess small bowel recovery.

31. Brain tumours

D. **A 50-year-old woman with insidious-onset unilateral deafness on Weber's testing sound is louder contralaterally and with some ipsilateral reduced facial sensation**

The 65-year-old man most likely has presbycusis – reduced ability to hear high-frequency sounds with ageing. The 40-year-old woman with insidious unilateral deafness experiences sound louder on the affected side with Weber's testing – this is indicative of conductive rather than sensorineural deafness. There is also no other neurology mentioned. Regarding cerebellopontine angle tumours, the most common is the vestibular schwannoma (formerly known as the misleading "acoustic neuroma"), representing 80% thereof. The café-au-lait spots of the 30-year-old woman are indicative of neurofibromatosis type 1 (von Recklinghausen disease). This neurocutaneous syndrome is not in fact associated with vestibular schwannomas, whereas neurofibromatosis type 2 is. This syndrome typically presents with bilateral vestibular schwannomas, and rarely are café-au-lait spots a feature. Furthermore, facial weakness coming on over days with no other neurological deficit is not typical of a cerebellopontine angle lesion. Cranial nerves V, VII and VIII are typically involved in a cerebellopontine angle lesion – although facial weakness can often be absent despite marked compression. The man with bilateral facial weakness, nasal voice and swallowing difficulty appears to have widespread involvement of the lower motor cranial nerves – a bulbar palsy. His age and the speed of onset should raise suspicion of motor neurone disease. That leaves the 50-year-old woman with sensorineural deafness of insidious onset (Weber's louder contralaterally) and some reduced ipsilateral facial numbness (cranial nerve V involvement). The unilateral sensorineural deafness of slow onset is typical and is due to the slow-growing benign tumour compressing cranial nerve VIII. Vertigo is uncommon, as compensatory mechanisms can act over the long period. If the tumour grows larger than 2 cm in diameter, the cranial nerve V can be compressed, leading to pain, numbness and paraesthesia. Cerebellar symptoms such as ataxia and nystagmus may appear with very large tumours, and rarely, fourth ventricle compression can give a raised intracranial pressure.

32. Chest injury

A. **Beck's triad**

Beck's triad of (1) muffled heart sounds, (2) engorged neck veins and (3) hypotension indicate acute cardiac tamponade, in this case caused by a stab wound to the myocardium. The resultant haemorrhage fills the fibrous pericardium, reducing the space available for the heart to fill in systole. Diastolic volume is therefore steadily reduced as the haemorrhage continues, leading to a possibly fatal reduction in cardiac output. Pericardiocentesis is required acutely: a cannula is inserted to the left of the xiphisternum under cardiac monitoring (an electrocardiogram [ECG] change can indicate contact with the myocardium, i.e. that you've gone too far). Upon penetrating the pericardium, the blood can be drained and cardiac output restored. Beck also performed the first defibrillation in 1947 with equipment made to his design by his friend James Rand Jr, who also invented the electric shaver (under the Remington brand).

Kussmaul's sign is a raised jugular venous pressure (JVP) upon inspiration that falls in expiration and is seen in constrictive pericarditis. This does not happen reliably in acute cardiac tamponade, where neck veins remain distended throughout respiration. Kussmaul also first described the deep, slow and laboured breathing pattern that occurs late in the severe metabolic acidosis of diabetic ketoacidosis and renal failure.

A Stokes–Adams attack is syncope, with or without seizures, resulting from a transiently reduced cardiac output and can occur in any position and during sleep. Virchow's triad describes the thrombotic risk factors of hypercoagulability, venous stasis and endothelial injury.

Claude Beck, American cardiac surgeon (1894-1971)

Adolph Kussmaul, German physician (1822-1902)

33. Complications of hepatitis infection

C. Hepatocellular carcinoma

Chronic hepatitis B and C infections are associated with a significantly increased risk of hepatocellular carcinoma. Hepatocellular carcinoma is also an important consequence of liver cirrhosis and should be suspected in any patient with rapid development of weight loss on a background of cirrhosis. Within the general population the prevalence is 4 per 100,000 people. Investigations include serum alpha-fetoprotein, followed by either liver biopsy or computed tomography (CT) imaging. Surgical resection, radiofrequency and/or microwave ablation are possible for early-stage cancers. The prognosis is extremely poor for non-resectable tumours, and there is a 20% 5-year survival rate for operable tumours.

34. Conn's syndrome

C. Conn's syndrome causes excess aldosterone, the vasoconstriction from which leads to hypertension

Primary hyperaldosteronism is a cause of excess aldosterone secretion, which leads to increased serum sodium concentration irrespective of plasma renin concentration. It is a secondary cause of hypertension. (Of note: 50% of patients with Conn's syndrome are normokalaemic, so a normal potassium does not rule out the diagnosis.) It is Conn's syndrome if this is due to an aldosterone-secreting adrenal adenoma. This is the cause in <5% of cases; 70% are caused by bilateral idiopathic adrenal hyperplasia. The increased plasma sodium causes fluid retention, which leads to hypertension. Aldosterone is secreted by the adrenal glands and stimulates the kidneys to retain sodium and excrete more potassium. The diuretic spironolactone is an aldosterone antagonist that will retain potassium and shed sodium and hence cause diuresis. Loop diuretics like furosemide and bumetanide cause a much more profound diuresis by inhibiting sodium, potassium and chloride reabsorption, and hence potassium is lost.

35. Dysphagia

E. Oesophageal carcinoma

The man has several risk factors and "red flags" for carcinoma: significant weight loss, significant pack-year smoking history and dysphagia for solids. All these factors warrant an urgent 2-week referral for oesophageal carcinoma and endoscopic evaluation. Histologically, oesophageal carcinoma may be adenocarcinoma or squamous, with the trend to increasing numbers of adenocarcinomas over the traditional squamous. Histology also varies with location in the oesophagus. The major risk factors for oesophageal carcinoma include smoking and alcohol intake, as well as the presence of Barrett's oesophagus in adenocarcinoma. Epstein–Barr virus infection has also been linked to the aetiology of the disease. Oesophageal carcinoma often presents late in the course of the illness and hence holds a relatively poor prognosis. Treatment may be with radical surgery, radiotherapy or palliative stenting. The 5-year survival rate for resectable tumours is 10–25%.

36. Diagnosis of chest infection

C. *Legionella* spp.

This patient has severe community-acquired pneumonia (CURB-65 score is already 3 due to confusion, raised urea and age >65, without the knowledge of the blood pressure [BP] and heart rate [HR]). *Legionella* species can cause a severe bilateral pneumonia in middle to old age. It can be associated with local epidemics originating in cooling towers or water reservoirs. It is a Gram-negative aerobic bacterium. Urinary antigen testing can quickly diagnose and thus guide antibiotic therapy. *Escherichia coli* is more commonly causative of hospital-acquired pneumonia. An antigen test for viral causes of pneumonia would be clinically useless. *Mycoplasma pneumoniae* is more common in children and young adults.

The condition is known as Legionnaires' disease, as it was first recognised as causing an outbreak of pneumonia in a group of elderly men attending an American Legion (war veteran) conference in Philadelphia.

37. Diagnosis of cough

A. **Asthma**

Asthma is characterised by chronic airway inflammation and increased airway hyper-responsiveness leading to symptoms of wheeze, cough, chest tightness and dyspnoea. The features that increase the probability of asthma include:

1. More than one of the following symptoms: wheeze, cough, breathlessness and chest tightness – particularly if symptoms are worse at night and in the early morning; if symptoms occur in response to exercise, allergen exposure and cold air; or if symptoms occur after taking aspirin and beta-blockers
2. History of atopic disorder
3. Family history of asthma and/or atopic disorder
4. Widespread wheeze on auscultation
5. Otherwise unexplained low FEV_1 or peak expiratory flow (PEF; historical or serial readings)
6. Otherwise unexplained peripheral blood eosinophilia

A diagnosis of asthma is made by compatible clinical history with either/or:

1. $FEV_1 \geq 15\%$ (and 200 mL) increase following administration of a bronchodilator/trial of corticosteroids
2. >20% diurnal variation on ≥ 3 days in a week for 2 weeks on PEF diary
3. $FEV_1 \geq 15\%$ decrease after 6 minutes of exercise

Scottish Intercollegiate Guidelines Network (SIGN)

British Guideline of the Management of Asthma

London: British Thoracic Society 2008

38. Diagnosis of Cushing's syndrome

B. **Computed tomography (CT) of the adrenals**

The history suggests that this patient has adrenocorticotropic hormone (ACTH)–dependent Cushing's syndrome. Compared to ACTH-secreting pituitary tumours, ACTH-secreting ectopic tumours do not have residual negative feedback sensitivity to cortisol. Ectopic ACTH-secreting tumour is associated with very high ACTH and cortisol levels. A high ACTH level is associated with marked skin pigmentation, which is described by the patient as "tanned". A high cortisol level could cause profound hypokalaemia, severe muscle wasting and severe hyperglycaemia. An overnight low-dose dexamethasone suppression test, 48-hour high-dose dexamethasone suppression test and plasma ACTH test are used in the workup of the diagnosis of ACTH-dependent Cushing's syndrome. Computed tomography

(CT) of the chest is useful in detecting a possible bronchial origin of an ACTH-secreting tumour.

39. Diagnosis of neurological dysfunction

C. Motor neurone disease

The lack of cerebellar involvement, optic neuritis, eye movement disorder, lack of sensory involvement and the patient's age all go against a diagnosis of multiple sclerosis (MS). However, in older patients, MS is more likely to be primary progressive, so the lack of relapses does not go against it necessarily. The patient seems to have a mixture of upper and lower motor neurone weakness in the limbs, which could go with cervical spondylosis, syringomyelia or motor neurone disease (MND) or MND-like syndromes. The lack of sensory involvement points to MND or an MND-like syndrome. Syringomyelia starts with the lack of pain sensation in the arms before giving more prominent lower motor neurone weakness in the arms and then later upper motor neurone weakness in the legs. Cervical spondylosis commonly presents with shooting pains in a dermatomal distribution in the arms and would give upper motor neurone but not lower motor neurone signs in the legs. Brisk reflexes in a wasted limb is a classic sign for MND and comes from a combination of upper and lower motor neurone loss with an intact sensory input into the reflex loop. The patient's age is classic (>50 years) and progression swift, with patients typically dying 3–5 years from onset. Patients with MND are at risk of developing frontotemporal dementia too. Retroviruses such as HIV and polio (on a more limited scale, both in terms of affected limbs and worldwide disease burden with the introduction of improved sanitation and vaccines) can cause lower and upper motor neurone loss with sparing of sensory neurones, and thus HIV can give an MND-like syndrome. However, this patient does not have a travel history or medical history to make us consider this.

40. Diagnosis of rheumatoid arthritis

B. Anti-CCP antibodies

Antineutrophil cytoplasmic antibody (ANCA) is associated with small vessel vasculitides such as Wegener's granulomatosis (cytoplasmic ANCA+) and Churg–Strauss syndrome (perinuclear ANCA+). Anti-centromere antibodies are associated with limited cutaneous systemic sclerosis. Rheumatoid factor is the traditional screening test for rheumatoid arthritis; however, it is only positive in 70–80% of cases, and it is present in many other autoimmune diseases, i.e. it lacks specificity. It is also present in 25% of persons over age 65 who do not have rheumatoid arthritis. Soft tissue swelling may be seen on X-ray of the hands but this is non-specific, and bony erosions are a late change that would not be expected in this case.

Anti-cyclic citrullinated peptide (anti-CCP) antibody testing is 98% sensitive and far more specific to rheumatoid arthritis and therefore represents a superior test. However, it is important that diagnosis is made using the American College of Rheumatology (ACR) criteria using clinical findings in addition to antibody tests.

41. Diagnosis of skin lesions

D. Rosacea

The distribution (cheeks, nose) may be described as "malar", and the areas are all exposed to the sunlight. This makes a rash worsened by sunlight more likely. Whilst it is a typical distribution for the rash of systemic lupus erythematosus, this is a fairly rare condition. It also does not usually present with papules and pustules. Some patients with rosacea can develop rhinophyma too. Dermatomyositis is an extremely rare condition that can feature a heliotropic or sun-sensitive rash, as well as Gottron's papules on the hand and linear erythema on the dorsum of the hand, along with an inflammatory proximal myositis. The qualities of the rash described do not sound like eczema, which is typically dry and itchy and does not feature papules or pustules. Acne vulgaris does feature papules and pustules, usually on the face as well as the upper back and shoulders, but this typically affects those in the throes of puberty. Rosacea affects those in middle age, more typically women, and is more common than systemic lupus erythematosus and does feature papules and pustules on a background of erythematous skin. The first-line treatment is oral tetracyclines (such as lymecycline).

Malar, from Latin *mala* = cheekbone

Rosacea, from Latin *rosacea* = rose-coloured

42. Electrocardiogram

B. Occasional P-waves are failing to conduct through and trigger QRS complexes

First-degree heart block is a prolonged P-R interval (>0.2 second). The P-wave is suffering a constant delay as it passes via the atrioventricular node (AVN). Second-degree heart block comes in two forms: either a P-R delay that increases with time until a beat is missed (Mobitz type 1 or Wenckebach block) or beats are missed in a ratio, i.e. every third beat (Mobitz type 2). Second-degree block is more serious and is best treated with pacing. Complete heart block (third degree) is more serious again and requires permanent pacing. Beats are driven by a pacing focus distal to the AVN (normally at a bradycardic pace), and the P-wave is therefore dissociated from the QRS complexes. These patients are vulnerable to Stokes–Adams attacks and are treated with a pacemaker. ST-segment elevation indicates ischaemia, and irregularly irregular complexes are a feature of atrial fibrillation.

Woldemar Mobitz, Russian physician (1889-1951)

Karel Frederik Wenckebach, Dutch cardiologist (1864-1940)

43. Emergency management

C. Intravenous lorazepam

In any situation it is essential that the patient's airway, breathing and circulation are intact before progressing to the management of any underlying condition. The first-line antiepileptic medication used in seizures is intravenous lorazepam. It is important to have full resuscitation equipment available when administering intravenous benzodiazepines since there is a risk of respiratory arrest. If intravenous access is not possible, alternative options include rectal diazepam or buccal midazolam. If the benzodiazepines fail to stop the seizure, an intravenous infusion of phenytoin should be started. If this fails, an anaesthetist should be called to initiate general anaesthesia.

44. Supraventricular tachycardia

A. Administer adenosine

Supraventricular tachycardias are often paroxysmal and can last from seconds to hours. They can be caused by coffee, alcohol and tobacco but are usually the result of atrioventricular node (AVN) re-entry tachycardia (dual pathways within the AVN) or Wolff–Parkinson–White syndrome (an accessory pathway outside of the AVN). The narrow-complex tachycardia can exhaust a heart and precipitate failure due to inadequate filling during diastole, leading to reduced cardiac output. The Valsalva manoeuvre and carotid sinus massage can end this arrhythmia, as can cardioverting with adenosine (a very short-acting AVN blocking agent). For adenosine to work, it must be administered promptly: intravenous injection over 2 seconds via a large-bore cannula. The patient should continue to receive cardiac monitoring, and the ward crash trolley should be close at hand, as excessive AVN delay can lead to arrest.

Antonio Maria Valsalva, Italian physician (1666-1723)

45. Syndrome of inappropriate ADH secretion

D. Urine osmolality 800 mOsm/kg, plasma osmolality 250 mOsm/kg

This question should be simple to work out from first principles. If the syndrome features *inappropriate* ADH secretion (SIADH), then the urine should be concentrated in the face of dilute plasma. By simple homeostatic principles, if the plasma is dilute, the urine should become more dilute in an attempt to concentrate the plasma. Option A, dilute urine with dilute plasma, could represent fluid overload. Option B, dilute urine with normal plasma concentration, could represent any cause of diuresis, which could become option C if the patient does not receive enough fluid intake! Option D shows concentrated urine but dilute plasma, consistent with SIADH. Option E shows concentrated urine with concentrated plasma, which is most likely due to dehydration.

46. Systemic lupus erythematosus

A. Acute pleuritis

Systemic lupus erythematosus (SLE) is a chronic multisystem connective tissue disease of unknown cause. Almost 90% of affected individuals are women, with a peak onset in the second and third decades. Patients present with myriad symptoms that could affect virtually every organ in the body. Constitutional symptoms such as fatigue, fever, and weight loss are present during the course of the disease, occurring in 50–100% of patients. Pleurisy, pleural effusion, pneumonitis, interstitial lung disease, pulmonary hypertension, and alveolar haemorrhage can all occur in SLE. In this case the presence of a friction rub and pleural effusion suggests the diagnosis of pleuritis. The pleural effusion in SLE is a mild exudate characterised by an elevation in pleural fluid low-dose heparin (LDH) but without signs of marked inflammation. Patients normally respond to therapy with non-steroidal anti-inflammatory drugs (NSAIDs), and moderate- to high-dose steroids are used if there is no response to NSAIDs within a few days.

47. Urinary frequency

D. Hyperosmolar hyperglycaemic state (HHS)

HHS is a condition characterised by severe hyperglycaemia (>30–50 mmol/L) without significant hyperketonaemia or acidosis. It usually affects older patients, of which many have undiagnosed diabetes or a past medical history of type 2 diabetes mellitus. In HHS the circulating insulin is sufficient to prevent ketogenesis but insufficient to allow the peripheral uptake and metabolism of glucose. As such the patient does not become acidotic. The hyperglycaemia causes an osmotic diuresis that rapidly dehydrates the patient and produces an extremely high plasma osmolality. There is hyperosmolality (>320 mOsm/kg) with severe dehydration, and pre-renal uraemia is common. The conscious level is depressed when plasma osmolarity is high, and the result is coma. These patients are usually sensitive to insulin, and approximately 0.05–0.1 U/hour of insulin should be given initially. Excessive rates of fall of blood glucose (>5 mmol/hour) may be associated with cerebral oedema. Isotonic saline is given unless serum sodium exceeds

155 mmol/L, in which case 0.45% saline should be used. These patients are prothrombotic and therefore have a high risk of deep vein thrombosis. Thus prophylactic subcutaneous low-molecular-weight heparin is recommended. The mortality rate of HHS approaches 30%, which is likely to reflect the advanced age of many of the patients and the presence of underlying illness.

48. Wilson's disease

B. Ask the patient to come in for an urgent blood test

Wilson's disease is an autosomal recessive disease of copper metabolism. In health, copper is transported in the serum bound to caeruloplasmin and is excreted in the bile. In Wilson's disease there is a defect in copper metabolism so it is not excreted in the bile and instead accumulates in the tissues. This process suppresses the synthesis of caeruloplasmin, which allows unbound (free) copper to enter the circulation. The high levels of free serum copper accumulate in vital organs such as the liver (cirrhosis), eye (Kayser–Fleischer rings), kidney and basal ganglia of the brain (personality changes). If left untreated the patient is at risk of developing cirrhosis, renal tubular disease, neurological disease and neuropsychiatric complications. Patients with Wilson's disease have an elevated serum free copper, low serum caeruloplasmin, high urinary copper and high hepatic copper (via biopsy). Paradoxically, total serum copper is usually low.

Penicillamine is used in the treatment of Wilson's disease, as it chelates copper and other minerals and hence can prevent the deposition of copper into organs such as the liver and the central nervous system. Its use can reduce and help reverse pre-cirrhotic liver disease, although neurological damage is often less reversible. It binds to circulating copper and facilitates its excretion in the urine. There are serious side effects of penicillamine, and patients should be advised to report any sore throat, temperatures or bruising. These signs may indicate agranulocytosis and immunosuppression that needs to be identified early, the drug stopped and necessary action taken. Therefore, advising the patient to come in for an urgent blood test to look at the differential white cell count and the platelets would be the safest course of action. These severe reactions are dose related but can occur early in the start of treatment; therefore, regular blood testing is advisable following the commencement of penicillamine.

Samuel Alexander Wilson, British neurologist (1878-1937)

49. X-ray changes in osteoarthritis

C. Punched-out periarticular erosions

Osteoarthritis occurs when the articular cartilage has worn sufficiently to narrow the joint space and bring the bones together – increased friction and trauma between the bones cause the pain. Sclerosis and osteophytes are the bone's reaction to this increased friction and trauma, which threaten to damage the bone. Subchondral cysts may also be seen on X-rays in osteoarthritis. "Punched-out" periarticular erosions are more associated with gout.

50. Traveller's diarrhoea

B. *Escherichia coli*

E. coli infection, in particular enterotoxigenic *E. coli* (ETEC), can occur by spread through contaminated food and water supplies, and it is the most common cause of diarrhoea in the returning traveller. The other causes listed should be suspected if diarrhoea is prolonged or there are other features such as mucus or blood in the stools. In prolonged causes of diarrhoea, parasitic infection such as *Giardia* should be tested for. Treatment is by oral or intravenous rehydration, as *E. coli* gastroenteritis is a self-limiting condition. Patients should be educated about meticulous hand hygiene.

Index

For Product Safety Concerns and Information please contact our EU
representative GPSR@taylorandfrancis.com
Taylor & Francis Verlag GmbH, Kaufingerstraße 24, 80331 München, Germany

www.ingramcontent.com/pod-product-compliance
Lightning Source LLC
Chambersburg PA
CBHW060827170526
45158CB00001B/100